Lᴏsᴛ Cᴀɴʏᴏɴs ᴏғ ᴛʜᴇ Gʀᴇᴇɴ Rɪᴠᴇʀ

LOST CANYONS OF THE GREEN RIVER

THE STORY BEFORE FLAMING GORGE DAM

Roy Webb

THE UNIVERSITY OF UTAH PRESS

Salt Lake City

FOR JAY MUMMA, 1944–2011
A good friend on the river and off

The Defiance House Man colophon is a registered trademark
of the University of Utah Press. It is based upon a four-foot-tall,
Ancient Puebloan pictograph (late PIII) near Glen Canyon, Utah.

16 15 14 13 12   1 2 3 4 5

LIBRARY OF CONGRESS CATALOGING-IN-PUBLICATION DATA
Webb, Roy.
 Lost canyons of the Green River : the story before Flaming Gorge Dam /
Roy Webb.
    p. cm.
 Includes bibliographical references and index.
 ISBN 978-1-60781-179-4 (pbk. : alk. paper)
 1. Green River (Wyo.-Utah)—Description and travel. 2. Green River
(Wyo.-Utah)—History. I. Title.
 F767.G7W44 2012
 979.2'5—dc23
                        2011043355

All images, unless otherwise noted, are courtesy of Special Collections,
J. Willard Marriott Library, The University of Utah.

"The Fall of Cottonwoods" copyright 1998 by Terry Lynn Jarvie Gardner.
Originally published in *Settlements of Uintah County: Digging Deeper*
by Doris Karren Burton. Reprinted courtesy of Terry Lynn Jarvie Gardner.

Printed and bound by Sheridan Books, Inc., Ann Arbor, Michigan.

DISCLAIMER

All mileages referred to in the text and figures are based on Green River, Wyoming, as mile 0. The maps are for reference purposes only and should not be used for navigation.

The author and publisher are not responsible for the way you use this book, how you maintain personal safety, or the decisions you make while on waterways. You assume this responsibility when you choose to go on a waterway. Please do so thoughtfully and carefully.

CONTENTS

Acknowledgments   ix

Introduction   xiii

1   Before   3

2   Ranches and Badlands   25

3   Canyons and Rapids   45

4   Ashley Falls   67

5   The Rest of Red Canyon   85

6   The Dam   101

Requiem   129

Notes   139

Bibliography   151

Index   155

ACKNOWLEDGMENTS

It's a cliché to say that this book is like a river, but I'll do it anyway. The upper Green is composed of waters from several smaller streams; Black's Fork and Henry's Fork, Currant Creek, Sage Creek, Trail Creek, Allen Creek, Red Creek, and many others. Each adds its own distinct elements; one is a muddy badlands creek, another a clear mountain stream. All add up to the Green, a perfect example of synergy: the whole is greater than the sum of the parts. So it has been with this book. One person told me a story about growing up on a ranch now under water; another, long gone, kept a diary of a trip down the Green before World War II; yet another collected everything that had ever been written about the river and gave it to a library for future scholars. Like those different creeks and rivers, the many sources from which this book comes have also, I hope, become an example of synergy. Any errors of fact, omission, or interpretation are of course my own.

This book grew out of my first one, *If We Had A Boat*, first published by the University of Utah Press in 1986. In researching and writing that book I learned a great deal about the Green River as I traveled around to various archives and libraries and talked to a lot of old-timers who had grown up on the river. As I

worked on that first book, it dawned on me that the upper Green, now covered with hundreds of feet of water, had once been a place of rare beauty with a rich heritage and that not very much had been written about it. Some books described the area around the river, touching it now and then as gently as a breeze ruffles the surface, but that was all. I wanted to know more about it and ended up doing an epilogue to that book called "Tailwaves." It wasn't really much, just about a dozen descriptions of what the river had been like before 1956, when Flaming Gorge Dam was begun. I have done other books and articles and lectures in between—and some of the stories in this book have appeared in other forms, such as the *Outlaw Trail Journal*, *Utah Historical Quarterly*, and *Boatman's Quarterly Review*, and in three of my other books: *Call of the Colorado*; *Riverman: The Story of Bus Hatch*; and *High, Wide, and Handsome: The River Journals of Norman D. Nevills*. But this present book eventually grew from that epilogue. I've met so many wonderful people and worked in so many great archives and libraries since then that there is no way I can remember them in chronological order, so I'll just go as my memory moves me; this is by no means a measure of their importance.

My supervisor of some thirty years at

the University of Utah's J. Willard Marriott Library Special Collections, Dr. Gregory C. Thompson, has been unfailingly supportive of all my research on the Green River, to the point of letting me head off down the river or on a research fellowship for a month at a time. I owe Greg a lot for his support over the years. I'm also grateful to my wonderful staff in the Multimedia Archives—Lorraine, Krissy, Justin, and Molly—who took up the slack when I was gone for those aforementioned periods. Of my esteemed colleagues in the Special Collections Department, Walter Jones stands out not only because he's always been such a good friend but for his deep and broad interest in and knowledge of the history of Wyoming and the West. Kirk Baddley, University of Utah archivist, has added a great deal to my knowledge of the salvage surveys conducted by University scientists in the 1950s and 1960s.

Other archivists and librarians around the region also deserve acknowledgment: Ruth Lauritzen and her helpful staff in the Sweetwater County History Museum in Green River, Wyoming; the librarians at the Uintah County Library Regional History Center in Vernal, Utah, including Elaine Carr and Michele Fuller; my archival colleagues at the Utah State Historical Society: Dr. Phil Notorianni, Kent Powell, and Doug Misner; and the archivists at the Cline Library Special Collections and Archives Department of Northern Arizona University, especially Richard Quartaroli, whose knowledge of how our interests in the river overlap has led to many fruitful discoveries. Mark Gerber deserves a great deal of praise for volunteering to create the beautiful maps that add so much to the book. I never met the late Michael Johnson, a fine historian, but his excellent, comprehensive, yet engaging book *A History of Daggett County: A Modern Frontier* (an entry in the Utah Statehood Centennial county history series) was a great resource for details about the area I was studying. I especially want to show appreciation to the Huntington Library in San Marino, California, a private library that holds the collection of Otis Reeder "Dock" Marston. Dock was entranced with the Colorado River from his first venture onto its waters in 1942 and spent the rest of his life collecting every letter, journal, and photo he could find from anyone who went down the Colorado River. As a consequence, the Marston collection has become a Holy Grail of Green and Colorado River historians; thanks to curator Bill Frank, scholars are able to plumb the depths of what Dock so obsessively collected. I've spent several periods working in the Marston papers, culminating in a Wilbur R. Jacobs Fellowship that allowed me to spend a whole month—such bliss!—conducting research for this present book. My feeling that the Marston collection would be a treasure trove of knowledge about the Green River turned out to be correct, and much of this book is derived from what I learned during that wonderful month.

The community of river runners is a small one. I've been lucky enough to know many boaters and to hear their stories about the early days on the Green firsthand, around a campfire on a riverside beach or sitting on a cooler in a boating company warehouse. Among many, I'd especially like to thank Brad Dimock, Gaylord Staveley, Rich Quartaroli, Al and Alison Holland, Ken Sleight, Joan Nevills–Staveley, Kent Frost, Earl Perry, Don and Ted Hatch, and Bob and Richard Quist. I learned a great deal from some who were long past their river-running years when I met them, such as A. K. Reynolds, Mike Hallacy, and Bill Purdy. Others I never met personally, for they are long gone; but as archivists often do, I got to know them very well indeed through their books, diaries, and letters. Among these are Norman D. Nevills, Buzz Holmstrom, Ralf Woolley, Antoine de Seynes, and Ellsworth Kolb, who left such detailed accounts that I feel as if I'd been on the river with them.

Those who lived around the river were an amazing source of far more information and memories than could fit in this book. Keith Smith, whom I never met, left a charming book of reminiscences. Ellen Reynolds was one of the first outfitters on the river, along with her husband, A. K. Reynolds. Barbara Williams Amburn, who grew up on a ranch near the mouth of Henry's Fork, is so full of stories that she almost stumbles over them trying to get them out. She has preserved a treasure chest of Green River history. Terry Lynn Jarvie Gardner grew up along the river and kindly allowed me to reprint her poem "The Fall of Cottonwoods." One of the pleasures of this book has been getting to know these people and many others who have lived their lives in the area now flooded by Flaming Gorge Reservoir.

Two friends who helped me with this book in different ways left us while this work was in progress. One was my friend Robert W. Jones, whom I always called Bobby even though he was a bit older than me. I coaxed Bobby out onto the river only a couple of times, for roughing it for him was staying in anything less than a four-star hotel. Yet his comfortable home in Vernal, Utah, provided a welcome base for research and river trips on the Green and Yampa for years. On more than one occasion Bobby picked me up at some river warehouse on the outskirts of Vernal at the end of a trip, gave me a rum and orange juice, and made dinner while I told him about experiences that he really had no interest in duplicating. The other was my good friend Jay Mumma, with whom I worked for almost three decades at the Marriott Library. Jay—known to all for his terrible puns, always delivered with a big smile—and I did so many things together, from building a wooden frame and floor for my raft to running rivers. Once the raft was finished, before the varnish and light coat of river sand went on, we both signed it; those marks are still there to this day. We ran the Jordan River in Salt Lake City, spent frigid early spring nights on the Green waiting for the moon to rise, and canoed the Colorado. He was always willing to run a shuttle, to pick us up at the end of a trip, to bring a forgotten but vital piece of gear to a halfway point between home and launch. It was Jay who told me about seeing a magazine in the bathroom of a kayak shop in California open to an article I'd written, and we both laughed at the thought that I'd arrived as a writer. They were both good friends, and I'll always miss them both.

Finally there is my family: my wife, Becci, and my two daughters, Rachel and Sarah. Becci has always been there for me whenever I've come back, sunburned, scratched, and sandy from a river trip, and has supported me in all ways, for better or for worse. Rachel has always chosen her own path; Sarah has always wanted to help others choose theirs. Both were dipped into the Green River before they could crawl, and neither seems the worse for it. They are the best things I've ever done.

INTRODUCTION

Like one of my favorite writers—Ann Zwinger, the author of *Run, River, Run*, the best book ever written about the Green River—I was born by a river. In my case it was the San Juan River of the Four Corners region. My parents lived in the Shady Grove trailer court by the old San Juan River bridge in Farmington, New Mexico, and while it's true that I was actually born in the new county hospital across the bridge, we did live right on the other side of the river. No doubt one of my very first acts as a human, when I was a couple of days old, was to cross the San Juan on that bridge in my Dad's '52 Chevy Powerglide. We moved away when I was a baby, but in the course of following the oil we came back the summer before I went into the fourth grade, this time to a 1950s modest ranch house in a development right out of TV land, where all the streets had Spanish names: Camino Real, Camino Placer, Camino Largo. More importantly, it was on the point of land formed by the Animas and San Juan Rivers, on the south side of town. The Río de las Animas Perdidas (River of Lost Souls) came down from the foothills of the San Juan Mountains to the north. The San Juan ran east to west through cottonwood-lined bottoms across the southern part of the town; the two met just before the old bridge on the west end.

Just a quick bike ride down the block from our house was the edge of the tangled cottonwood bottoms along the north side of the San Juan. Across the river were towering sandstone cliffs that ran for miles, locally called the Bluffs. That marked the boundary of Dine-tah: Navajo land. We could never look at those cliffs across the river without a shiver; there we saw mystery, old legends, lost civilizations, scary stories of skin crawlers and witches and secret rituals. It was a great place to grow up. We rode our horses for hours in the sandy dry washes that led to either river, over juniper-covered hills. The river bottom by our house was a jungle of old cottonwoods, willows, swampy places, strange rustlings in the leaves, and if you went far enough, there it was: the San Juan. In the winter the water took on a strange translucent green, almost like turquoise, and you could make your way far out into the channel on ice-rimmed sandbars. But in the spring you could only stay on the shore and watch. The river swelled and turned brown, a muscular, impulsive flow of swirling currents filled with cottonwood logs and sometimes even whole trees. Summer and fall were best, when the river was low enough to wade into and the water was warm. All the neighborhood kids played army there, made bike jumps, shot BB guns, snuck out at night and met under a full moon. I've always said it was a perfect place to smoke a stolen cigarette, try a stolen beer, steal a kiss from a girl for the first time.

I moved away after high school, north to Vernal, Utah. It was actually a lot like Farmington in its landscape and feel: empty desert to the south (Ute lands), mountains to the north, sandstone and badlands and cottonwoods in between, a big river nearby. My adolescent fascination with the San Juan proved fickle; I transferred my affections to the Green River—love at first sight. I don't remember the first time I saw the Green. It must have been while crossing the bridge at Jensen, on one of those marathon midwinter expeditions to see my sister Guinn in Vernal. My father would drive straight through snow, fog, and mud, over unpaved roads; it took about three packs of Lucky Strikes to get there. Later I saw Split Mountain: I was about twelve when we went to the Dinosaur Quarry. After that I moved in and out of Vernal, went to college, dropped out of college, worked odd jobs here and there, went back to college, but the river was always there in the background. Whenever I had free time I would drive over to Rainbow Park or Split Mountain to visit it, like seeing a friend. Somehow I got into running rivers. I'm sure it had something to do with my nephew Rodger, my sister's oldest son; he and I grew up together. Rodger usually had some grand scheme that he would sell you on, and rivers happened to be one of them. I had turned into a backpacker by this time, hiking all over the

Uintas and Wind Rivers and down in southern Utah. I wasn't a purist; but river running seemed, I don't know, to require too much gear and too much work. Rodge persuaded me, however, and there we went.

My very first real river trip was on the Green below Flaming Gorge Dam about 1975. I was living in Salt Lake City then, enamored of a Mormon girl whose ward had an outing there. So I went along, more for her brown eyes and thick wavy hair than anything else. But once we got to the river I found myself distracted by the flowing water, and since the whole relationship with her wasn't going anywhere anyway, the river took my attention. I came back a while later with Rodge and our friend Bob in a little yellow raft—more a pool toy than a serious watercraft—for an overnight trip. After we were dropped off at the boat ramp, Flaming Gorge Dam loomed over us just upstream. We nervously blew up the boat, put our gear and food in big plastic garbage bags in the bottom, and pushed off. The river was icy, as it still is. As the air in the tubes cooled, the boat immediately softened. We weren't smart enough to stop and pump the tubes back up, so gallons of frigid water poured into the boat if we sat on the tubes. We sat on the floor instead, which wasn't much better and had the added disadvantage that we could barely see because we were sitting down so low. We paddled through a whole series of little rapids, which to our inexperienced eyes were raging cataracts, and camped overnight at Little Hole, in those days rarely visited. At the end of the trip, we had asked our friend Mike to pick us up "in Browns Park." None of us had ever been there, and we didn't know it was an almost uninhabited, forty-mile long valley traversed by only a single dirt road. But, after ducking under the Taylor Flats Bridge and walking along the road, we somehow found each another. That first overnight trip had been cold and scary and quick; from that day to this I have never stopped thinking about the Green River.

After that I started running rivers whenever I could get away. Over the next several years I did go back to that same stretch of river below the looming dam many times. It taught me a lot: how to row a boat in rapids, how to tie one up and how not to tie one up onshore, how to rig and bail, and what kind of oars to buy. I started running other rivers, but this was the place where I started writing about them. One last encounter before we move on: some years later I was doing an overnight trip there with Rodge and some other friends. By then I was an experienced and studly boater with a $273 Udisco raft from Sunset Sports (some friends called it a U-Fold-o but I called it a *Volksboot*) complete with a homemade wooden rowing frame and Mae West life jackets. We were just getting ready to go, but the boat ramp there is always busy. Along came a Mormon ward on an outing, with that same Mormon girl. There's always a certain measure of guilty satisfaction in meeting an old love when you are with your new one: the river had long since stolen any affection I might have felt for her wavy brown hair.

Later I spent a long winter at the Jarvie Ranch, at the end of Red Canyon and the beginning of Browns Park. Duward and Esther Campbell had bought the Jarvie Ranch in the 1960s and lived there until Duward died about 1970. After a few more years, Esther wanted to move to town, so the Nature Conservancy bought it to turn over to the Bureau of Land Management (BLM) as a historic site. After working in Dinosaur National Monument for a summer, I got a job as a winter GS-5 Park Tech for the BLM, in charge of the Jarvie Ranch as well as the north side of the river from Red Creek down to the Taylor place. That sounds grander than it was; I was totally out of my depth, having never lived in such a remote place and not being naturally handy with tools, unlike the traditional ranch dweller. If I hammer a nail straight without hurting myself I feel as if I'm doing well. But I managed not to burn down the house by luck and by drawing on help from the nearest neighbor, on a ranch about twelve miles away. I got there about a week before the Jonestown Massacre and heard about it on the Rock Springs country western station—the only station I could get. I thought to myself, "Maybe this is a good time to be up here." I lived in an old double-wide trailer; the only other residents were a cat named Stickerbush, some golden eagles who lived in an old cottonwood at the end of Jarvie's meadow, and the deer who would come into the yard and rub their antlers on the side of the trailer at dawn. They made a loud scraping noise that would catapult you out of a warm bed, no matter how many times you heard it. It was thirty miles to a paved road, another fifty miles to a town. The party-line phone worked unless it had snowed; "no phone, no lights, no motor car, not a single lux-ur-y."

But I did have one constant faithful companion: the Green River. It flowed a stone's throw from the back door of the trailer, just past a giant gnarled old silver maple tree. I spent many hours—days, really—walking along the river, sitting by it, watching it, talking to it. You can only read so much, only listen to Joni Mitchell albums so many times, and I got tired of writing in the multivolume journal I kept (and haven't looked at since). So there was always the river. It was constantly entertaining—more than that: intriguing. Just like the San Juan of my youth, it asked me questions: Where was it going? Where had it been? At the risk of sounding trite, the Green was alive. I got to know its moods, when Red Creek had flooded, when the ice was breaking up along the banks, when the geese were coming back. Very few people fished there—none, really, that winter, but I don't remember any even in the spring. Now, of course, the Jarvie Ranch is a developed and interpreted official historic site and that area is like a moving walkway at an airport, with cars and boats and trailers. But then it was pretty much all mine. I walked up to Red Creek Rapid sometimes, about four miles; and just about every day I climbed up the hill above the house for a view all over Browns Park and back up into Red Canyon.

You could say this book was born then, but it took some gestation. At one point in that lonely winter I was sent to Salt Lake City on an errand and for some reason stopped at the University of Utah to say hello to one of my former professors, Dr. Gregory C. Crampton, in his office in the old Annex. He graciously let me take up his time, babbling—for I was rather starved for conversation—about the Green and the ranch and Browns Park and John Jarvie and the river. Finally he stopped me and said in his cultured, erudite voice: "Why don't you write about this?" I stammered and I stuttered: "I could never . . . I'm not a writer . . ." He broke in again: "Of course you could. You were a good student and you wrote good papers. Write about this."

That conversation swirled around in my head like a stick in an eddy. When I finally made my way back to the university for another bout with the degree, I took a required senior seminar in history and wrote a sixty-page paper on the history of the Green River. I chose that class specifically because it was open ended: you could write about whatever you wanted. So I took Dr. Crampton's advice and wrote about what I knew: the Green River. I got an A. Somewhere in there I tired of oil-field and summer seasonal jobs and got a position indoors, in the Marriott Library. And I got married, which meant that I did indeed finish the degree and an additional one. I saw a little article in the newspaper around that same time reporting that the University of Utah Press was looking for manuscripts, so I sent them the history paper. They called me and said, "Let's talk about this." Out of that meeting—and with encouragement from the late Peggy Pace, my first editor—came my first book, *If We Had A Boat*, published in 1986.

The book you hold in your hands eventually grew from a short epilogue in *If We Had A Boat*. That afterthought ultimately came together with a lot of writing and reading and talking about the Green River since then—four other books, hundreds of articles, scores of lectures, weeks and months spent on the river, in boating company warehouses, and in pickup trucks going to and from the river—to create this book, just as rills and creeks and brooks combine to create a river. Like any river it was a long and sometimes "remarkable crooked" course to get here. Since 1986 I've been thinking about writing a book about the Green before Flaming Gorge Dam was built. So the present work is the culmination of a lifelong task I set myself, and I only hope that it's worthy of the river and the people who were as affected by it as I have been.

This book describes the course of the Green River from the town of Green River, Wyoming, through the open valley north of the Uinta Mountains, through Flaming Gorge, Horseshoe, Kingfisher, and Red Canyons, to the upper end of Browns Park and the Jarvie Ranch—a distance of about a hundred miles as the pikeminnow swims. I'll confess that I was sometimes tempted to wander off course and overflow my banks, like the Green in flood, into the deep and sometimes turbulent history surrounding the river valley or fetch up on

the obscure sandbars of geologic history. But those subjects are better left to other writers, so this book concentrates on just the river itself: how it appeared to travelers who floated down it and what it was like to camp under the cottonwoods near the Firehole Towers or pull up to the Holmes Ranch, swatting mosquitoes and meeting Mrs. Holmes for the first time, or scramble up on the boulders for your first nervous look at Ashley Falls, already anticipating the tug of the current as it grabs your oars. The Green is forever changed in this reach—as the old saying goes, "You can't get there from here." I've always collected river guidebooks, which stand in for the real thing when it's frozen over. Think of this book as a guidebook for a river you can no longer run.

Most of this reach has been inundated by Flaming Gorge Reservoir since 1963. Under the reservoir are the ghosts of ranches, corrals, and ferries as well as memories of every phase of American western history: Indians, trappers, soldiers, Mormons, homesteaders, ranchers, outlaws. Yet despite all that coming and going and striving and living and dying during 165 years of exploration, exploitation, settlement, and the construction of one of the largest dams in the United States, very little is known about the history of this particular section of one of the largest river systems in North America. The blank spaces on early maps with hardly any transition have become blank spaces that show only open water, not the meadows, ranches, towns, canyons, rapids, and forests that they once contained. The

Green River between the town of Green River, Wyoming, and Flaming Gorge Dam, some hundred miles downstream, remains in some ways just as unknown as it was when the first trappers ventured down it in boats made from buffalo hides so many years ago.

When the Glen Canyon Dam was authorized, large teams of archaeologists, historians, biologists, and other scientists were sent out to survey the cultural and natural heritage about to be lost to Lake Powell. The surveys produced shelves of documents, thousands of photographs, hundreds of feet of film, and dozens of scientific reports. In the ensuing years, scores of nonfiction books, articles, novels, documentaries, and memoirs of Glen Canyon have been produced, rhapsodizing about its lost beauty and the wonders once found along the Colorado River. Poems have been penned and songs have been composed, and environmentalists have launched serious campaigns to remove the dam. Glen Canyon has been eulogized as "The Place No One Knew."

As part of the Colorado River Storage Project, Flaming Gorge Dam was authorized and constructed at the same time as Glen Canyon Dam. Yet even though the canyons and valleys of the upper Green River were beautiful and full of human history, hardly a word was said when the gates of Flaming Gorge Dam were closed and the entire stretch of river, some hundred miles of valleys and canyons, was flooded and forever lost. This loss has not been commemorated in books, songs, films, or poems, and no environmentalists are praying for the removal of Flaming Gorge Dam. Flaming Gorge Reservoir, and the truncated stretch of Red Canyon below the dam, has become known as a blue-ribbon fishery, a playground for water skiers and boaters, an economic engine, and an impoundment to keep water away from the lower Colorado River Basin states. These days few realize or care about what lies beneath them; but a river once flowed where only power boats can be seen now, along the reach of the Green from Green River, Wyoming, to the middle of Red Canyon. Beneath those cold, clear waters, ranchers and farmers and families once lived, deer and elk and antelope and mountain lions and bears thrived, and tall cottonwoods leaned into the winds. Simply put, Glen Canyon was not the only "Place No One Knew."

LOST CANYONS OF THE GREEN RIVER

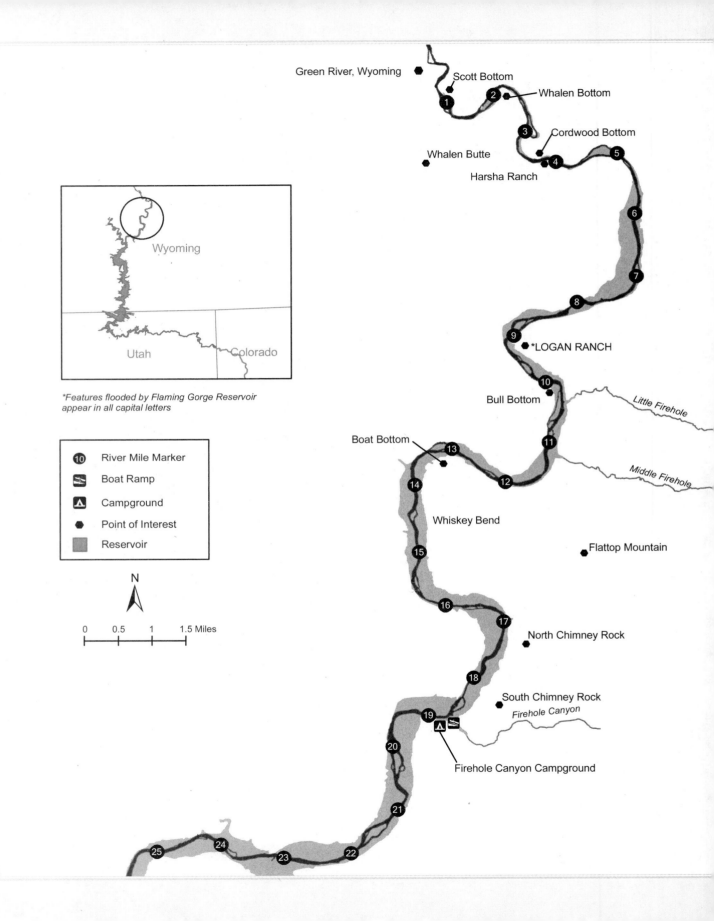

Green River, Wyoming

Scott Bottom

Whalen Bottom

1

2

Cordwood Bottom

Whalen Butte

3

5

4

Harsha Ranch

6

7

8

9   *LOGAN RANCH

Little Firehole

10

Bull Bottom

11

Middle Firehole

Boat Bottom

13

12

14

Whiskey Bend

15

Flattop Mountain

16

17

North Chimney Rock

18

South Chimney Rock

19   Firehole Canyon

20

Firehole Canyon Campground

21

25   24   23   22

*Features flooded by Flaming Gorge Reservoir
appear in all capital letters

Wyoming

Utah   Colorado

10   River Mile Marker

Boat Ramp

Campground

Point of Interest

Reservoir

N

0   0.5   1   1.5 Miles

BEFORE

The course of the Green and Colorado is but little known, and that little derived from vague report. Three hundred miles of its lower part, as it approaches the Gulf of California, is reported to be smooth and tranquil; but its upper part is manifestly broken into many falls and rapids. From many descriptions of trappers, it is probable that in its foaming course among its lofty precipices, it presents many scenes of wild grandeur; and though offering many temptations and often discussed, no trappers have been found bold enough to undertake a voyage which has so certain a prospect of a fatal termination.

—JOHN CHARLES FRÉMONT (1843)

The River and the Land

The Green is one of the major rivers of the West and the major stem of the Colorado. It rises in the Wind River Mountains of central Wyoming and flows for 730 miles before it reaches the confluence with the Colorado in what is now Canyonlands National Park. The upper Green first flows north then makes a great bend to the south and continues on that course, with a few exceptions, for the rest of its length. From the town of Green River, Wyoming, it flows through open country and badlands and then in canyons until it reaches Browns Park, about a hundred miles below Green River. The open reach was about 65 miles long: the river meandered in sweeping curves first through plains and later through badland country of buttes and cliffs set away from it. The river bottoms in the open country and badlands were lined with cottonwood and willow trees, while the open country away from the river was mostly sagebrush. James Clyman, who first came into the country with Jedediah Smith in 1824, was back again twenty years later. He described the open country above the canyons in terms that still apply after more than a hundred years:

> In about two hours ride we came to green river a beautiful clear crystal Stream about one hundred yards wide & nearly bel– low [*sic*] deep to our Horses running East of S. through a sandy parched dry coun– try but little of it clothed with grass. Some groves of Shrubby cotton wood growing on its banks. After crossing we rode down the vally [*sic*] of this stream about 6 miles East of South over the Bluffs 12 miles to Black fork which Stream likewise runs into Seetskadee. About 20 miles east of whare [*sic*] our trail struck it. All the high ground dry & dusty & covered with the Eternal Sage which can live without rain from June until October on a clean pure gran– ite gravel.[1]

About sixty miles below Green River, the river cut through a series of hogback ridges that parallel the Uinta Mountains, thrust up by the same forces that created them. After a few more miles of open country, the river enters one of the more dramatic river canyons to be found anywhere: Flaming Gorge. In the canyons, great Douglas firs and ponderosa pines came right down to the water's edge; the only openings were at the mouth of side streams like Sheep Creek and Carter Creek, marked by clear, cold, mountain brooks full of cutthroat trout.[2] Flaming Gorge, Horseshoe, and

Kingfisher Canyons are each hardly ten miles in length, but they make up in variety what they lack in distance.[3] Flaming Gorge is a dramatic curving entrance into the Uinta Mountains. Its color comes from the bright red Chinle and Moenkopi Formations. After only a mile and a half, the river enters Horseshoe Canyon, a big bend reminiscent of a horseshoe. It differs dramatically from Flaming Gorge, being cut through muted gray sandstones and mudstones. At the end of the bend, barely two miles in length, the river passes an open area called Nielson's Flat then enters Kingfisher Canyon, named for the many birds of that species seen there. This is yet another short canyon, cut through the Weber Sandstone. This buff-colored formation creates dramatic cliffs that tower over the river. The river runs north and south, so the cliffs tend to block out the sun for most of the day, giving a gloomy effect. After Beehive Point, a steep cliff with so many cliff-swallow nests that it reminded early explorers of a beehive, the river passes Hideout Flat, rumored to be a haunt of outlaw gangs and horse thieves. A hidden trail came down Hideout Canyon and crossed the river at this point, taking advantage of the shallow river in this short opening in the canyons.[4]

Just below Hideout Flat the river turned east and entered Red Canyon, so named for the deep red color of the Uinta Mountain Quartzite through which it was cut. Red Canyon was not only the longest of this series of canyons (almost thirty miles) but the first place a traveler on the river would encounter real rapids.

Above the canyons were no rapids, only gravel bars and strainers caused by cottonwood falling into the river. Even in Flaming Gorge, Horseshoe, and Kingfisher Canyons, the softer rocks meant that the river could wear away anything washed in from a side canyon (the most frequent cause of rapids), creating only small riffles, such as the one off Beehive Point. But in Red Canyon, once boulders of the dense, resistant, Uinta Mountain Quartzite fell or were deposited in the river by a side canyon flood, they tended to stay there. River runners know that harder rock means harder rapids, and Red Canyon proved this rule. At the mouth of every little side canyon was a rapid of varying degrees of difficulty, including some that were treacherous, such as Skull Creek, or dramatic, like Ashley Falls, or even deadly, like Red Creek. Red Canyon ends just a few miles below Red Creek Rapid (about 100 miles below the town of Green River), as the river flows quietly into Browns Park, as if weary from the struggles with the hard rocks above.

At this point it should be said that before the Green River was tamed by Fontenelle and Flaming Gorge Dams it was not the limpid stream that today attracts fly fishers and Boy Scouts to the truncated stretches below both dams. It was muddy, muscular, unpredictable; fed by the melting snows of the Wind River and Uinta Mountains, it could rise quickly and reach a flood level of over 25,000 cubic feet per second (cfs).[5] The peak flood usually started in late May and was over by the middle of June. These floods could wash away buildings, fences, or ferries and could undercut the banks and drop whole groves of cottonwood trees into the river. Flooding also made it almost impossible to cross the river without a sturdy, stable boat from just about anywhere below the town of Green River. At other times of the year the river could practically dry up or even freeze over in the winter. The annual floods made the rapids in Red Canyon seem considerably different at various times of the year, and all that water trying to enter the narrow Flaming Gorge caused whirlpools and eddies, which gave rise to the legend of the dreaded but mythical "Green River Suck" (of which more later). In the low-water seasons, the rapids were frequent and rocky, with tight channels—"technical," in today's river parlance; but when the big floods came, the smaller rapids washed out and were covered up. The bigger ones, though, such as Skull Creek, Ashley Falls, and Red Creek, just got bigger, becoming roaring cataracts with crashing waves and spray. No wonder early river runners feared the rapids in Red Canyon, no matter what the season.

Wildlife

Like the rest of North America before the coming of the Europeans and their guns, railroads, and livestock, the country around the Green was teeming with wildlife; as Bill Purdy put it, there were so few people that the whole area "belonged to the animals." The plains were home to buffalo, deer, and antelope, while there were elk, moose, and bighorn

sheep in the mountains. Purdy often saw elk swimming the river during their migrations. One winter in the 1950s Purdy and a Forest Ranger crossed the Green on the ice, climbed to a hill overlooking Little Hole, and counted over a thousand deer.[6] The deer, elk, and bighorn sheep were preyed upon by coyotes, wolves, mountain lions, and black and grizzly bears. Grizzlies were often called "white bears" because of their silver fur. They were especially feared, because before they were driven into the mountain wilderness—and to the edge of extinction—they liked to live in the willow and cottonwood bottoms along the river.

Another feature of the open country was herds of wild horses that roamed the hills and river bottoms. Many smaller mammals occupied the bottom of the warm-blooded fauna, such as foxes, marmots, and prairie dogs, while multitudes of beaver lived along the river. Beaver, otters, and muskrats attracted the first fur trappers. Buffalo flourished around the valley of the Green until the 1830s; huge herds were commonly sighted by the earliest travelers to cross the river. Virtually every early party that crossed the plains would linger around the Green to "make meat," shooting numerous buffalo and drying the meat for the arduous passage across the Utah and Nevada deserts and the Sierras. The Bidwell-Bartleson party of California-bound emigrants met mountain men on the banks of the Green who claimed to have eaten nothing but buffalo meat for ten years and wanted to trade for bacon and flour.

By the 1840s, however, the buffalo had succumbed to hunting and were no longer to be found along the Green River.

The river was a major flyway for waterfowl, so at the right times of year thousands of geese, ducks, cranes, swans, herons, pelicans, and other wading and swimming birds could be seen, especially along the cottonwood bottoms. Other types of birds were likewise plentiful, as noted by Ellsworth Kolb in 1909:

> [In September] . . . in Kingfisher Canyon were a few of the fish-catching birds from which the canyon took its name. There were many of the tireless cliff-swallows scattered all through these canyons, wheeling and darting, ever on the wing. These, with the noisy crested jays, an occasional "camp robber," the little nuthatches, the cheerful canyon wren with his rollicking song, the happy water-ouzel, "kill-deer," and road-runners.[7]

Large soaring and predatory birds such as golden and bald eagles, ospreys, red-tailed and other kinds of hawks, falcons, and the ubiquitous vultures were also common. Sadly, the buffalo were not the only wildlife hunted to extinction; Dick Dunham writes in a letter to Otis Marston in 1977: "One thing I wasn't aware of, though probably you've known about, was that up until the early [1870s] there were large numbers of swans on the Green from Flaming Gorge to Swallow Canyon. A few nested at the mouth of Lodore. They were vigorously hunted and by the '80s they were all gone . . . Hook and Galloway were swan hunters."[8]

One inhabitant that did not excite any admiration was the mosquito, clouds of which rose from the river bottoms in the open country after the spring floods began to recede. These afflicted wildlife and domestic animals, river runners, and ranchers alike for several months in the spring and summer and were frequently noted by everyone who lived in or traveled through the area. In 1962 archaeologist Kent Day reported that during the course of a survey of the area south of Manila the crew was "driven back to the higher terraces by swarms of mosquitoes. A mere plural is insufficient for the numbers that live in the sage and marshy flats . . . I have never seen such aggressive and immodest insects."[9]

The fish were also much different than those that the modern traveler finds. Because of the dam, the reservoir now contains mostly introduced game fish—pike, bass, walleye, and others—with trout in the cold, clear stretch of Red Canyon below Flaming Gorge Dam. In the days before the dam, though, the muddy, warmer river was home to many fish that are now all but extinct. These were ancient bottom-feeding fish, such as squawfish, now known as the Colorado pike minnow but then called "white salmon" or "Colorado salmon"; boneytail and humpback chubs; and razorback suckers, known locally as "buffalo chubs." They traveled up and down the Green to spawn. The fish could grow to enormous sizes, with tales told of squawfish three and even four feet long being caught that weighed up to thirty-five pounds. Even though they were full of tiny bones, all of these fish were eagerly consumed by Native Americans and the early settlers alike.[10] As early as 1841, a member of the Bartleson-Bidwell party of emigrants camped on the banks of the Green noted: "We caught some good fish called chubs."[11] These were not the only fish in the river; trout were native to the side streams. Some of them would have been found in the main channel. After the area began to be settled, carp, catfish, and many other species of fish were introduced through one means or another and soon thrived.

Long before History

There is evidence of very early Paleoindians in the area around the upper Green River almost as soon as the glaciers in the Wind River and Uinta Mountains melted, when great herds of mammoths, mastodons, camels, giant short-faced bears, bison, and sabertooth cats roamed the plains, followed by the hunters. One site of a mammoth kill has been found to the north, near the Bighorn River in central Wyoming, and sites in the Pine Springs area to the east of the Green River date as far back as 13,000 years ago. Fire pits, knife blades, and projectile points have been found in southwestern Wyoming, demonstrating that people of the Clovis, Folsom, and Plano archaeological cultures both traveled through the area around the Green and lived along its banks.

Given the abundance of game, they had little reason to stray too far from the river; but as an area was hunted out, they would move to new grounds. Along the way they would harvest roots, berries, and seasonal shoots, but game remained the major portion of their diet. Of course we have no way of knowing how they viewed the river, whether they ever ventured onto it, or how they crossed it, but it must have been a big part of their lives. Based on sites throughout southwestern Wyoming, it would seem that aboriginal groups more or less permanently occupied the region, for the same reasons that later Native Americans as well as more recent residents did: wood, water, and game. The area has a combination of natural resources and climate that makes it a good place to settle.[12]

The Paleoindian period was followed by the Archaic about 11,000 BP (before present), marked by two technological shifts: milling stones and coiled baskets. These indicate that people were now staying in an area longer to exploit concentrations of food. The mano and metate, both milling stones, were used to grind hard seeds that earlier hunters had ignored because they required so much processing. The baskets were used for cooking stews and gruels by placing hot stones into them and likewise showed that the inhabitants now had a much broader diet. By this time too the megafauna was beginning to die out; while hunting was still an important part of their lifestyle, the people began to follow smaller game such as bighorn sheep, deer, rabbits, antelope, and many littler animals. Waterfowl and fish taken from the river were also a part of their diet—another reason to stay close to the Green. The first repetitive use of the landscape began to occur at this time, with intermittent reuse of hunting camps, storage caches, and rock art areas. The late Archaic, from about 5,000 to 3,000 years ago, was a time of growth in population. By the end of the Archaic period, the entire group no longer moved camp to obtain resources such as food, tools, and raw materials, which were brought back to the group, leading to the first small villages.[13]

Archaic groups inhabited the Green River country now covered by Flaming Gorge Reservoir for an incredibly long time, over ten millennia. During that period they roamed the banks of the Green, hunting, gathering, and sporadically reusing areas with the best resources. But other ancient peoples were also on the move around the end of the Archaic. Bows and arrows were introduced in the area north of the Colorado River around AD 100–200.

The archaeological culture known as Basketmaker II, which originated in the Four Corners region, crossed the Colorado River and probably followed the corridor of the Green River from the south, reaching what we know as the Uinta Basin about 2,000 years ago. During their journeys the Basketmaker II people encountered the indigenous Archaic peoples, and the two populations mingled. This created what would come to be known as the Fremont culture, named for the Fremont River in central Utah. Evidence of the Fremont can

be found throughout the interior West, from the Great Basin of eastern Nevada to western Colorado, from southern Wyoming all the way to the Colorado River in southern Utah, but the earliest identifiable Fremont sites are in the Uinta Basin.

The Uinta Mountains, forming the northern boundary of the Uinta Basin, are not much of a barrier. The northward movement over the mountains continued into the land that 2,000 years later would become Flaming Gorge Reservoir. The people moving up from the south brought a whole new way of life with them, including, most importantly, farming. From the Mesoamerican cultures far to the south they had learned to cultivate corn, beans, and squash. The Steinaker Gap area, just to the south of the upper Green River basin, contains the earliest evidence of irrigation in the Fremont area. The inhabitants still foraged for wild plants and hunted for game, but by AD 250 more than half their calories came from maize. Fremont people lived in small pithouses clustered in extended family or clan groups, farmed fertile patches of land at the mouths of canyons, and stored their crops in small storage cists or in granaries set high in inaccessible canyon walls, including Red Canyon.

The land just north of the Uinta Mountains that would eventually be flooded by Flaming Gorge Reservoir contained many small Fremont sites. During the brief salvage survey completed while the dam was being built, archaeologists from the University of Utah identified over 120 such sites. These ranged from storage cists in Red Canyon near the dam site to small temporary camps in sand dunes and large lithic scatters (areas where stone tools were made or repaired). In some places the ground was literally covered with chips. One of the favorite pastimes of ranchers and other Anglos who lived in the area was hunting arrowheads. Because of the annual flooding, it is unlikely that people of the Fremont culture farmed right along the Green River—why put so much work into a field that would surely be lost to inundation every year? But they did use small patches of sandy soil in side canyons and draws. Such farming sites were even found in the depths of Red Canyon, at the mouths of Trail Creek and Jarvies Canyon.

Other artifacts characteristic of the Fremont were distinctive footwear (both moccasins and sandals), small figurines made of clay, and gray utility pottery. These argued for a semisedentary lifestyle, since nomadic people would not have wanted to carry pottery or heavy milling stones around. Rock art first appeared during the Archaic period, but the Fremont people are best known for their magnificent rock art, found all over the intermountain West. Rock art panels are especially widespread and beautiful in the area just south of the Uinta Mountains, but they were also found on the northern foothills of the mountains. One such rock art site, near Henry's Fork, featured a "300 foot long discontinuous petroglyph panel."[14] These panels were adorned with representations of bighorn sheep, elk, and other large mammals;

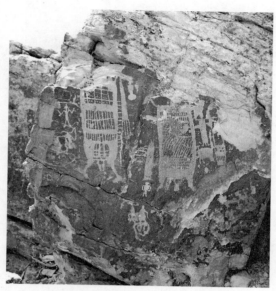

Petroglyphs near Henry's Fork.

geometric figures such as spirals, lines, and irregular patterns of dots that could represent maps; and elaborate human figures. Known as trapezoidal anthropomorphs for their wide shoulders, narrow waists, and stick arms and legs, the human figures were often decorated with elaborate headdresses and necklaces. Those found in the Uinta Basin sometimes showed what look like human heads being held like trophies. A humpbacked flute player along the Green River near the mouth of the Yampa is thought to indicate a direct influence from Mesoamerica. Shield figures are also common north of the Uintas, which some archaeologists have argued shows influence from the Great Plains to the east. Alas, many of these sites were near the Green River and were covered when the waters of Flaming Gorge Reservoir rose in the 1960s.[15]

Seeds-Kee-Dee Agie

The Fremont people famously and mysteriously vanished around the middle of the fourteenth century, probably victims of their own success. Their skills at farming allowed the population to rise beyond sustainable levels. After a change in climate and precipitation patterns, such as occurred about AD 950, farming became impossible. In fact, just as the earliest traces of the Fremont are found in the Uinta Basin, the earliest evidence of abandonment is also found there. The Fremont people did not just completely vanish from one day to the next; archeologists have found indications that many of them simply returned to a hunting-gathering lifestyle when farming was no longer possible. Ute legends tell of encounters with people who must have been Fremont when they first entered the Uinta Basin in the 1400s. But by and large the Fremont people were gone from the upper Green River basin by AD 1000. They were replaced by Numic speakers such as the Shoshones and the Utes, who began moving into the region around the same time.

By the time the Spanish began to land far to the south, around 1500, the various tribal groups had sorted themselves out. The area from the Wind River Mountains to the northern slopes of the Uintas was occupied by the Eastern Shoshones, who lived a nomadic hunter-gatherer lifestyle, much as their ancestors had done. There were two main bands: the Mountain Sheep Eaters, who lived around what is now Yellowstone National Park, and the Buffalo Eaters, who traveled on a seasonal cycle between the Uinta Mountains and the Wind River Mountains, throughout the basin of the Green River. The Shoshones were also known as the Snakes, for the waving motion they used to describe themselves in sign language; the people of the band that lived in the area now inundated by Flaming Gorge Reservoir were known as the Kohogues or Green River Snakes. That said, it's an oddity of history that the name for the Green commonly ascribed to the Shoshones, Seeds-Kee-Dee Agie (Prairie Hen River), appears to be a Crow name. *Agie* is "river" in the Crow language; the Shoshones apparently called the river Ka'na, meaning "Bitterroot," because of the abundance of those edible plants in the valley. The Utes, on the other side of the Uintas, referred to the Green as Pah-Na-Cuits (Bigger River).[16]

Like the ancient peoples before them, the Snakes had little reason to leave the valley of the Green River, for the surrounding area was teeming with game of all kinds. Buffalo, elk, deer, antelope, waterfowl, fish in the river itself, and many other kinds of wildlife, along with abundant edible plant resources, provided a comfortable living for the Eastern Shoshones. As in the case of most of the plains and mountain Indians, we have no evidence that they ever traveled on the river itself, but naturally they had to cross it to get back and forth to their hunting grounds. All of the fords of the Green River later used by trappers, immigrants, Mormons, and gold-seekers had long been used by the Shoshones. When the water was too high to ford the river, they used a bull-boat to get across, a small craft made of buffalo skins stretched over a wooden frame. Like the horse and numerous other things, the technique was borrowed from their neighbors on the plains.

Even before the Shoshones obtained horses in the 1700s, they were active traders and travelers, but horses revolutionized their lifestyle as it had so many others. With the horse, the Shoshones could roam far afield, hunting the buffalo still found around the Green until about the 1830s, trading or fighting with their neighbors such as the Crows, the Utes, and the Bannocks. Indians that lived even farther afield, such as the Blackfeet, Gros Ventres, and Nez Perces to the north, the Sioux and Arapahos to the east, and even the Navajos to the south, would occasionally make forays into the Shoshone lands. The Shoshones would likewise travel far afield for trading or war. In 1826 James Ohio Pattie, a peripatetic trapper and traveler, encountered a large band of Shoshones "clad in buffalo robes, equipped with muskets, and provided with horse and mule transport, on the Little Colorado [River], in Navajo country." Furthermore, they told Pattie that they had recently fought a battle with a company of French trappers on the headwaters of the Platte River, in Colorado.[17]

By the dawn of the fur trade era in the early nineteenth century, the Shoshones had become a powerful tribe numbering about three thousand individuals. Warren Angus Ferris, a trapper who visited a Shoshone village in 1830, left a detailed account of his visit:

> Their village consisted of about one hundred and fifty lodges, and probably contained above four hundred fighting men. The lodges were placed close to each other, and taken together had much the appearance of a military camp. I strolled through it with a friend, to gratify my curiosity, as to their domestic manners. We were obliged to carry clubs to beat off the numerous dogs, that were constantly annoying us by barking, and trying to bite our legs. Crowds of . . . children followed us from lodge to lodge, at each of which were seen . . . industrious women, employed in dressing skins, cutting meat into thin strips for drying, gathering fuel, cooking, or otherwise engaged in domestic labour. At every lodge, was a rack or frame, constructed of poles tied together, forming a platform, covered over with half-dried meat, which was curing over a slow fire.[18]

Besides Sacajawea, the most famous Shoshone was their leader Washakie, born to a Flathead father and a Shoshone mother in 1804. His father was killed by the Blackfeet when Washakie was a boy. After wandering for days, Washakie and his mother found refuge with the Lemhis, a branch of the Shoshones who lived along the Snake River in eastern Idaho. By the fur trade era in the 1820s, he

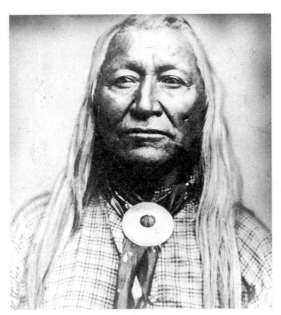

Washakie, chief of the Shoshones.

had settled with the Eastern Shoshones and become a famous warrior, fighting in many battles with their implacable enemies, the Crows or Absarokas, the Blackfeet, and the Arapahos and Sioux of the plains. Washakie had a prominent scar on his face from a fight that he wore with pride for the rest of his life. His skills in battle and his wise council soon made him the head of the tribe, and he remained the leader of the Eastern Shoshones until his death in 1900. During the heyday of the fur trade, Washakie and his band would often participate in the annual rendezvous, many of which were held on the banks of the Green River. They would announce their arrival by a thundering charge of hundreds of "hideously painted," screaming warriors, terrifying those traders or visitors not

used to this display.[19] Washakie was welcome at the rendezvous because he purposely maintained good relations with the whites, even helping them regain horses that had been stolen by other tribes. Jim Bridger was a particular friend of Washakie and even married one of his daughters. After the Mormons came into the Green River basin in 1847, Washakie met with their representatives and traded gifts with Brigham Young. He refused to be drawn into the Utah War in 1857–58, despite the entreaties and blandishments of the soldiers sent to quell the Mormon "rebellion."

At the height of their power the Shoshones were wealthy and secure; but like all other Native Americans, they did not benefit from their contacts with the white settlers. Unlike many Indian leaders, however, Washakie could see that what the future held was not good. Realizing that the white settlers would take whatever land they wanted, in 1863 he and other Shoshone leaders negotiated a peace treaty that laid out the boundaries of the Shoshone lands and provided for annuities; in return, the Shoshones agreed not to attack settlers, army posts, emigrant trains, stagecoaches, or telegraph crews. They held strictly to that agreement and subsequent treaties. Even during the upheavals of the 1870s the Shoshones remained at peace with the white settlers; a band of Shoshones even fought with Gen. George Crook against their ancient enemy, the Sioux, at the Battle of the Rosebud in June 1876. Eventually, though, Washakie decided that the only way in which the Eastern Shoshones could continue to exist was to remove themselves totally from the areas settled by whites. Another treaty, known as the Treaty of Fort Bridger, was signed there in 1868. Uncle Jack Robinson, another retired trapper and long-time friend of Washakie, acted as interpreter. The treaty formally established the Wind River Reservation on the east side of the Wind River Mountains. The Shoshones still hunted and traveled in their old ancestral lands; but after Treaty of Fort Bridger they could no longer claim the valley of the upper Green River as their own.

"A Wicked, Swearing Company of Men"

The earliest American explorers, Meriwether Lewis and William Clark and the later Astorians, passed to the north of the Green River, but they knew about the Green, which they called the "Spanish River," because the territory to the south was all claimed by Spain.[20] Within a decade of Lewis and Clark, American fur trappers started to move south from the upper Missouri River, driven out by the British and the relentlessly hostile Blackfeet Indians. The Snake River Expeditions of the Hudson's Bay Company, led by Donald MacKenzie and Peter Skene Ogden, explored the upper Green from about 1818 to 1825. Their goal was to trap out the beaver in order to create a "fur desert," thereby depriving the American trappers of any reason to come there. It was a forlorn hope, because numerous trappers from as far away as New Mexico and Missouri had already heard of the quantity and quality of the beaver

to be found along the Green and were on their way. Accordingly, businessman William Henry Ashley of St. Joseph, Missouri, sensing an opportunity, decided to enter the fur trade. In March 1822 he placed an advertisement in the *Missouri Republican*: "To enterprising young men. The subscriber wishes to engage one hundred young men to ascend the Missouri River to its source, there to be employed for one, two, or three years."[21] The men who answered the ad—who became known as the "Ashley Hundred"—included some of the most famous names in American history, such as Jedediah Smith, David Jackson, Jim Bridger, the Sublette brothers, Moses "Black" Harris, James Clyman, and many others.

Ashley formed a trapping brigade of these men and set off for the fur country. After a few disastrous false starts on the upper Missouri, he decided to shift his focus to the Green River. Ashley "came to the Shetkeedee" near the present Fontenelle Reservoir in April 1825 and set about not only trapping but exploring.[22] He split his party into four groups: Zacharias Ham led a party to the west; Thomas Fitzpatrick set out to the south, along the banks of the Green to the foothills of the Uintas; and James Clyman was sent north to the Wind River Mountains. Ashley, with the remaining seven men, set off down the Green in bullboats.

Ashley had another idea: instead of marching back and forth between Missouri and the fur country every year, the trapper brigades would winter in the mountains and meet at a "place of Randavouse [*sic*]" somewhere along the river to turn over their furs, get new supplies, and share information about the trapping season.[23] Ashley found his spot near the mouth of what he called Randavouse Creek (which we know as Henry's Fork) and cached his extra goods there, although the mosquitoes were so thick there that he later moved some miles up that creek. Proceeding down the Green, Ashley and his men had little difficulties in the open country above the Uintas, even in their ungainly craft; these were men from Missouri and Ohio, for whom travel by river had been a way of life for generations. Once they entered the canyons, however, they were more cautious—and with good reason. On Sunday, May 3, they came to their first real rapids:

> [T]he navigation became difficult and dangerous, the river being remarkably crooked, with more or less rapids every mile, caused by rocks which had fallen from the sides of the mountain, many of which rise above the surface of the water and required our greatest exertions to avoid them. At 20 miles from our last camp the roaring and agitated state of the water a short distance before us indicated a fall or some other obstruction of considerable magnitude . . . It proved to be a perpendicular fall of ten or twelve feet produce[d] by large fragments of rocks which had fallen from the [mountain] and settled in the river extending entirely across its channel and forming an impregnable barrier to

the passage of loaded watercraft. We were therefore obliged to unload our boats of their cargoes and pass them empty over the falls by means of long cords which we had provided for such purposes.[24]

While his men were portaging the supplies and lining the boats around the rocks, Ashley found a spot on the left wall and painted "ASHLEY 1825" in large black letters; the rapid was forever after known as Ashley Falls. A few days later, on May 5, after navigating several more rapids, the little party entered Browns Park and thus passed outside the scope of this book.

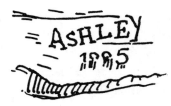

Ashley inscription at Ashley Falls, taken by Dellenbaugh in 1871. *From Frederick S. Dellenbaugh, The Romance of the Colorado River, 112*

The valley of the Green River remained a center for the fur trade throughout its brief but colorful history; indeed, most of the rendezvous were held near the Green, and some of the most famous incidents in the history of the mountain men swirled around the river. Many of the mountain men who survived were transients; they trapped, whooped it up at the Rendezvous, fought or traded with the Indians, and then moved on to California or Oregon or returned to the "States." Ashley himself spent only one season in the trade before selling his company to Jedediah Smith, David Jackson,

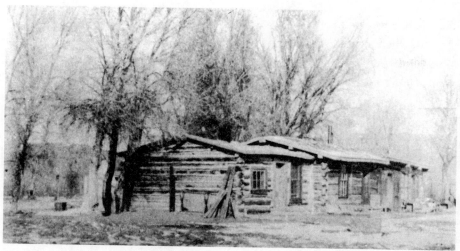
"Uncle Jack" Robinson's cabin on Henry's Fork.

and William Sublette and retiring to Missouri to begin a career in politics. But even after the trade began to die out in the late 1830s, when beaver hats were no longer in style, a number of the trappers took up other pursuits and stayed around the Green River, marrying Indian wives and settling down in the lush bottomlands. One who did so was Jim Bridger, who built several trading posts on the upper reaches of Black's Fork, in partnership with Henry Fraeb and—after Fraeb was killed by the Sioux in 1841—with Louis Vasquez.

Another former mountain man who settled in the country that would become Flaming Gorge Reservoir was "Uncle Jack" Robinson, who came to trap but stayed around the upper Green River for the rest of his life. Robinson was "tall, large, active fellow with a dapper moustache. He was honest, jolly, slouchy, dirty, seldom sober."[25] When the demand for fur collapsed in the 1840s, Robinson, like

several others, shifted to livestock trading. Around the same time, emigration to Oregon began to increase. Traveling the Oregon Trail was as hard on livestock as it was on the emigrants, and Robinson would trade one good horse, mule, or ox for two broken-down ones. After a few months' rest with good grazing, the animals were ready to be sold or traded once again. Robinson also had a trading post in Browns Park and spent part of his time living in a skin lodge with one of his Indian wives, Marook. Among his many residences was a cabin at the mouth of Henry's Fork that he built in 1836, which still exists and is one of the oldest structures in Utah.[26] Robinson was a great friend of Washakie and helped to negotiate the Treaty of Fort Bridger, as noted above. Uncle Jack died in 1882, long after the era of the mountain men was over, and was buried in the Fort Bridger cemetery.

Even though the fur trade was gone and the

mountain men had moved on to other pursuits by the 1840s, their legacy lives on along the upper Green River. Many names still on the landscape—Ham's Fork, for Zacharias Ham; Black's Fork, for Daniel Black, another of Ashley's men; Smith's Fork, for Jedediah Smith; and Henry's Fork, named for Ashley's partner Andrew Henry, among others—reflect the wild days of the mountain men, the fur trade, and the rendezvous.

If We Had a Boat

On July 23, 1841, on the banks of the Green River near the Sweetwater crossings, occurred one of those convergences of the past and the present beloved by historians. A party of trappers and some Shoshones under Henry Fraeb—"a wicked, swearing company of men," according to one witness—met with John Bartleson and John Bidwell.[27] These two men were the leaders of the first party of emigrants to try to take wagons across the continent on what would soon become the Oregon Trail. The emigrants were looking for information about the journey ahead, buffalo robes for the cold nights, and fresh horses—their own horses were worn out from the arduous trail. The trappers were after powder, shot, tobacco, and other supplies, especially the liquor that some members of the emigrant party had brought along to trade. The trappers bought up "the greater part, if not all" of the supply of whiskey and, after camping together for a day, went their separate ways.[28] Several members of the emigrant party left at

that point: some returned to the States, while others wanted to trap. They split further at Fort Hall, with a number of them taking the easier route to Oregon. Bartleson and Bidwell, who had brought boat-building tools so they could float to California if their wagons could not get through, finally struggled across Utah and Nevada and over the Sierras to California.[29] Fraeb was killed during a pitched battle with Cheyenne, Sioux, and Arapaho Indians in what is now Routt County, Colorado, shortly after this meeting.

The trails followed by the settlers passed to the north, crossing the Green near the Sweetwater River in the area now covered by Fontenelle Reservoir. As the flood of settlers grew, so did the need for ferries across the Green. Many of those ferries were operated by former mountain men, seeking a new trade now that beaver was no longer profitable. The legendary Jim Baker—friend of both Jim Bridger and Kit Carson and one of the survivors of Henry Fraeb's last fight with the Sioux in August 1841—opened a trading post on Henry's Fork in 1839, married one of Washakie's daughters, and for several years operated a ferry across the Green. As late as 1869 John Wesley Powell, camped just above Flaming Gorge, wrote about Baker:

> For many years this valley has been the home of mountaineers, who were originally hunters and trappers, living with the Indians. Most of them have one or more Indian wives. They no longer roam with

the nomadic tribes in pursuit of buckskin or beaver, but have accumulated herds of cattle and horses, and consider themselves quite well to do. Some of them have built cabins; others still live in lodges. [Jim] Baker is one of the most famous of these men, and from our point of view we can see his lodge, three or four miles up the river.[30]

But emigrants to Oregon and California were not the only travelers who needed a reliable way across the river. In 1847 the first party of Mormons crossed the Green headed for the new Zion that they hoped to establish in the valley of the Great Salt Lake. Their tale has been told so often that it need not be repeated here. Despite establishing a few small settlements nearby, they had only a passing influence on the parts of the river valley now covered by Flaming Gorge Reservoir. They eventually controlled Fort Bridger on Black's Fork and built Fort Supply on Smith's Fork. During the Utah War of 1857, the soldiers stranded at the site of Fort Bridger ran out of feed for their animals and moved them to Henry's Fork for pasture. But the sphere of Mormon influence was west and north of the valley of the Green itself.

For the most part, then, the great migrations on the Oregon and Mormon Trails bypassed the Green River valley between what would become Green River, Wyoming, and the Uinta Mountains. But at least a few parties looked at the smooth river flowing south, remembered

tales heard along the trail of the river coming out somewhere in California, and thought: "If we had a boat . . ." One such traveler who left a record was William Lewis Manly, an adventurous young man from Vermont. By 1849 he had already been knocking around the country for a few years and had just about decided to head for Oregon when he heard about gold in California. Joining a wagon train in Iowa, he reached the Sweetwater crossing of the Green late in the season. There Manly and the other drivers learned to their dismay that Mr. Dallas, the leader of the train planned to winter over in Salt Lake City and could not afford to pay them, so they would be on their own. Along the way they had fallen in with a troop of U.S. Dragoons who were on their way to Oregon. The surgeon of the dragoons was a well-traveled and well-read man who told them that he had learned the river they were on came out somewhere on the California coast. That was enough for Manly and six companions, who found an old abandoned ferry boat, dug it out, and decided to quit the wagon train and head for California the easy way, by river.

At first all went well. The river was smooth and tranquil, they found game in the cottonwood bottoms, and Manly and the others wondered why people would stare at the back end of an ox for months when they could just float down the Green in a leisurely fashion: "[I]t looked as if we were taking the most sensible way to get to the Pacific, and we almost wondered that everyone was so blind as not to see it as we did. . . . [W]e commenced to move down the river with ease and comfort, feeling much happier than we would had we been going toward Salt Lake with the prospect of wintering there."[31]

One day Manly and his party passed an Indian camp (probably at the mouth of Henry's Fork). The Indians came out and waved to them to come ashore, but they pressed on. The Indians might have been trying to tell Manly something, for on the fifth day the travelers' pleasant mood soured when they rounded a corner and the river seemed to disappear:

> [T]he boat came around a small angle in the stream, and all at once there seemed to be a higher, steeper range of mountains, right across the valley. The boys thought the river was coming to a rather sudden end . . . and for the life of me I could not say they were not right, for there was no way in sight for it to go. I remember while looking over a map the military men had, I found a place named Brown's Hole, and I told the boys I guessed we were elected to go on foot to California after all, for I did not propose to follow the river down any sort of hole into any mountain. We were floating directly toward a perpendicular cliff, and I could not see any hole anywhere, nor any other place where it could go.[32]

This was of course the entrance to Flaming Gorge, and while Manly and his men might have felt some measure of relief that the river did not indeed disappear down a hole and they would not be forced to strike off on foot, the abrupt change in scenery must have been unsettling. Much more cautiously, they entered the deep, gloomy canyons, finding that their relaxing journey had turned into something entirely different. As travelers familiar with navigating across open country, they must have noticed that they were now heading southeast, away from California. But by now they were committed; they had little choice but to carry on. At one point they saw a cottonwood tree with the marks of an axe on it and seized on that for some small comfort. Acting on the same impulse, once when they stopped to rest Manly climbed up on the cliff wall and painted his name, "CAPT W. L. MANLY, U.S.A.," on the canyon wall with a mixture of gunpowder and grease.[33]

Just below that spot Manly and his men came to Ashley Falls. As they were portaging their awkward craft around the rocks Manly noticed the name painted on the left wall; at least some white men had come this way! But shortly afterward their real troubles began. At another obstruction in the channel, they tried to get the ferryboat around the rocks. It got away from them and was swept up against the boulders in the channel, pinned there by the current. "We could no more hope to move it than we could move the rock itself," Manly wrote. Fortunately they had already unloaded all their supplies and baggage, but now they were well and truly stuck. But these were men used to hardship and to living by their wits; looking at the tall pine trees that lined the

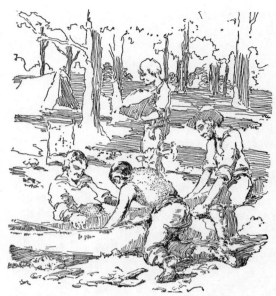

Manly and his men making dugout canoes, Red Canyon, 1849.

canyon walls, they decided that they could make dugout canoes to continue their journey. Chopping down two of the largest, they set to work, and "never let the axes rest night or day" until they had had fashioned two canoes, which they tied together side by side as a kind of catamaran. They quickly realized that there was not enough room for all of them, so they found more pines, and once again the canyon resounded to the sound of axes. With two of these vessels, they were finally able to resume their journey.[34]

Manly makes no mention of Red Creek Rapid, near the end of Red Canyon; by this time all the rapids in Red Canyon had probably started to blend together. Just before coming into Browns Park, he did remark on what was no doubt foremost on his mind, food:

"This rapid rate soon brought us out of the high mountains and into a narrow valley where the stream became more moderate in its speed and we floated along easily enough. In a little while after we struck this slack water, as we were rounding a point, I saw on a sand bar in the river five or six elk, standing and looking at us with much curiosity."[35]

Manly and a couple of his companions landed with their guns, stalked the elk, and killed two of them. The bull elk, he noted, "was a monster. Rogers, who was a butcher, said he would weigh five hundred or six hundred pounds. The [antlers] were fully six feet long, and by placing [them] on the ground, point downwards, one could walk under the skull between them." They stayed up all night drying the meat, which "made the finest kind of food, fit for an epicure," before continuing on to further adventures in the Canyon of Lodore and beyond.[36]

Hell on Wheels

The building of the transcontinental railroad was one of the greatest accomplishments of any age. Less than fifty years after the Ashley days and less than five years after the great cataclysm of the American Civil War, the nation was being spanned by steel rails that would reduce journeys like Ashley's and Manly's to a matter of days instead of months. As the rails were being laid, small towns sprung up to supply the workers and take advantage of the money to be made by selling lots or whiskey or whatever else might be needed. They

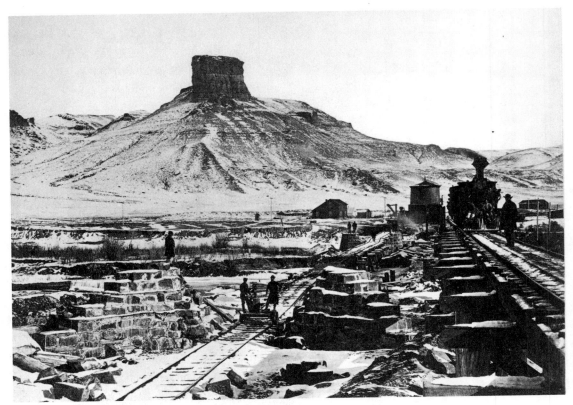

Construction of railroad near Green River, Wyoming, 1868. *Courtesy Library of Congress*

were generally rough places, generically called "hell on wheels," because they moved with the advancing railroad. One such town was Green River City, incorporated in 1868, as the Union Pacific was building a bridge over the Green River. The Union Pacific originally said that Green River City was to be a division point. But after disputes with squatters, including H. M. "Theodore" Hook, the former mayor of Cheyenne, and Jake Fields, owner of a saloon and general store, the railroad moved the division point to Bryan, twelve miles west, on Black's Fork. Green River City shriveled up and would

have become a ghost town if Black's Fork had not dried up a few years later. The trains needed a reliable water supply, so the division point was moved back to Green River (which had by then dropped the "City").

When John Wesley Powell shipped his boats to Green River in May 1869, he found only a few shanties and the Jake Fields store still hanging on. Some of Powell's men had gotten there before him; while waiting they found refreshment at the Fields saloon, as Jack Sumner, one of Powell's crew noted: "[We] tried to drink all the whiskey there was in town. The

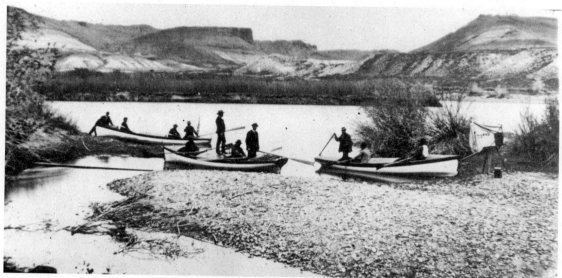

Powell launch, 1871.

result was a failure, as Jake Fields persisted in making it faster than we could drink it."[37] Naturally, Powell's upcoming expedition down the Green River was the talk of the small town, exciting the interest of everyone, including Theodore Hook, of whom more later.

With the coming of the railroad, great changes were in store for the valley of the upper Green River. The days when the Shoshones could hunt buffalo on the sage plains and the mountain men could trap beaver in the canyons were long gone. Now that people could get to Green River City, the empty lands along the river would begin to fill with ranches, homesteads, and families. Instead of the honking of thousands of geese, the river would hear the sound of a steamboat whistle.

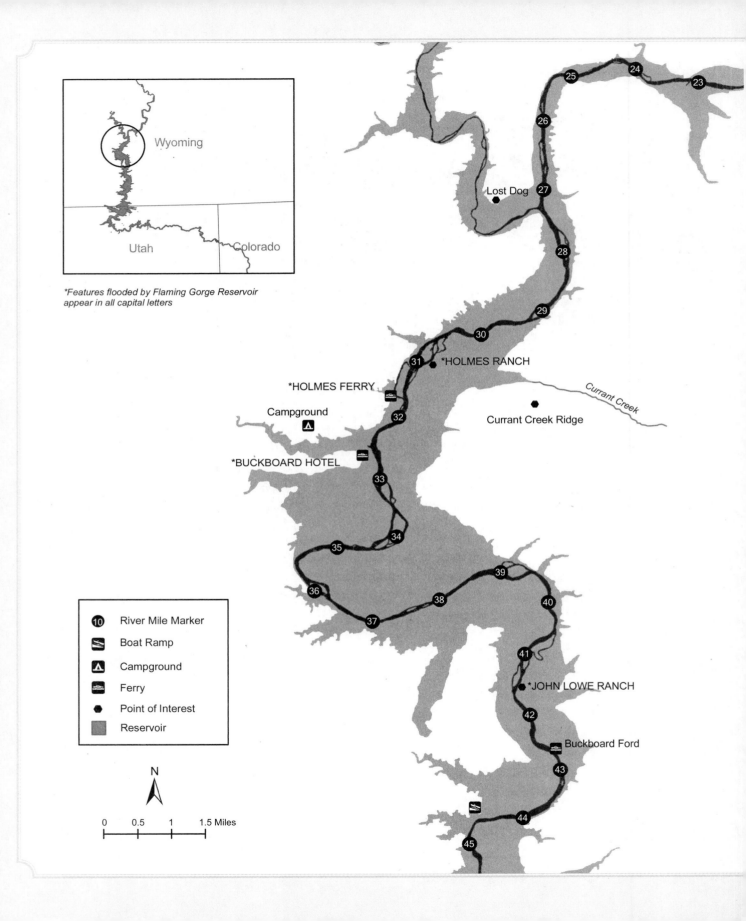

Wyoming

Utah   Colorado

*Features flooded by Flaming Gorge Reservoir
appear in all capital letters*

Lost Dog

*HOLMES RANCH

*HOLMES FERRY

Campground

Currant Creek

Currant Creek Ridge

*BUCKBOARD HOTEL

*JOHN LOWE RANCH

Buckboard Ford

River Mile Marker

Boat Ramp

Campground

Ferry

Point of Interest

Reservoir

N

0   0.5   1   1.5 Miles

RANCHES AND BADLANDS

Since leaving the basin and entering the valley of Green River, a remarkable change in the face of the country is apparent. Instead of the disturbed and upheaved rocks which characterize that region, flat tables or terraces of horizontal strata of green and blue sand and clay, and sandy conglomerate, or agglutinated sand, now form the principal feature of the country, standing alone, like island buttes, amid the barren plains, or forming escarpments which alternately impinge upon the banks of the winding streams. These tables, which extend from the rim of the basin to the South Pass, and thence to Brown's Hole, on Green River, are apparently the result of a deposit in still water. The layers are of various thicknesses from one foot to that of a knife blade, and the hills are fast wearing away under the influence of the wind and rain. The whole country looks as if it had, at one time, been the bottom of a vast lake, which bursting its barrier at Brown's Hole, had been suddenly drained of a portion of its waters, leaving well-defined marks of the extent of the recession upon the sides of these isolated buttes. As the channels became worn by the passage of the water through the outlet into Green River, another sudden depression followed, and the same operation was repeated at still a lower level.

—Capt. Howard Stansbury (1849)

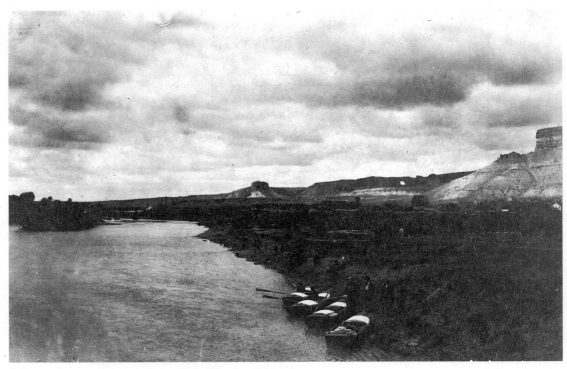

Galloway-Stone party launch, Green River, Wyoming, September 1909.

Before setting off down the river, it would be well to say a few words about launches from Green River, Wyoming. The first two voyages on the Green that we know about—those of William Ashley in 1825 and William Manly in 1849—left from the point where the Oregon, California, and Mormon trails crossed the Green, about 25 miles upriver from the present town. The first and one of the best-known expeditions to start from the town of Green River, of course, was that of John Wesley Powell, who chose a small island just downstream from the railroad bridge to set up his first camp and prepare his boats and equipment for the journey. Both of his expeditions, in 1869 and again in 1871, left from the same place. It was such a good spot (far enough from town to discourage pilferage of equipment but close enough to make it easy to get to stores for last-minute supplies) that many others followed Powell's lead; the Galloway-Stone expedition of 1909, the Kolb brothers two years later, and the United States Geological Survey (USGS) surveyors in 1922.

The most obvious reason for choosing this site was ease of access to the railroad: all of these parties shipped their boats by rail to Green River, Wyoming. They could unload their boats from the railcar then float

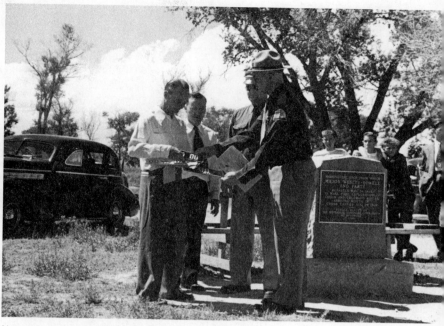

Norm Nevills launch ceremony, Green River, Wyoming, June 1947.

them downriver about a mile to Expedition Island. The Todd-Page party in 1926 left from the same place simply because the boats they purchased from the USGS were stored at the railyard. By the 1930s, however, trucks had become more common. Boats could now be hauled down the dirt road toward Linwood, so more people started launching from farther downstream—usually at the mouth of Henry's Fork, where Keith Smith's ferry road provided easy access to the river, or at Hideout Flat—to avoid the miles of flat water with its wind and mosquitoes. In 1938 the French kayakers launched from a hidden spot a few miles downstream from Green River because they were unsure whether their voyage required an official permit and did not

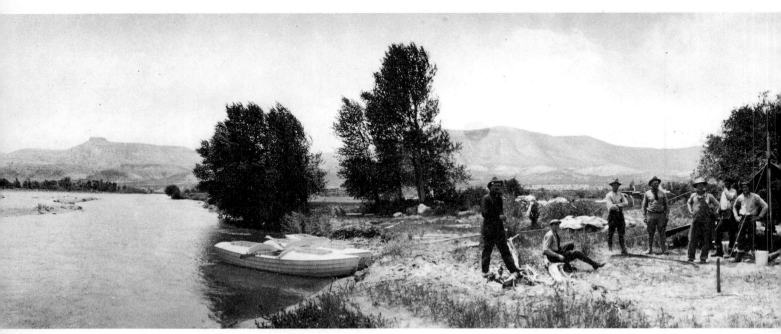

USGS party camped at Scott Bottom, 1922.

want to be stopped by authorities before they got on the river. While planning the expedition, Bernard de Colmont had written to Miner Tillotson, the superintendent of Grand Canyon National Park, asking if they needed a permit to run the river. Tillotson told Bernard that river running was so dangerous that they would have to post a $10,000 bond to cover the cost of the rescue expedition that would surely have to save them. After that, the French kayakers were leery of anyone who wore a badge or uniform or seemed official and generally tried to keep quiet about their journey.[1]

One person who always launched from Green River was Norman Nevills, not because of any real ease of access but because it gave him greater opportunities for publicity. Nevills was constantly looking for good press about his river trips; so when he decided to run the upper Green the first time in 1940, he contacted Adrian Reynolds, the owner of the local newspaper, the *Green River Star*. Reynolds was eager to oblige, because it would provide good copy for his adopted hometown. When Nevills came back to Green River for another trip in 1947, he and Reynolds concocted a publicity stunt that pulled out all the stops. Reynolds invited the governors of Wyoming and Utah to attend; Neither governor attended, but they did send representatives who brought official license plates from each state, which Nevills proudly affixed to his boat, the *WEN*.[2] A big crowd gathered to hear speeches and earnest pronouncements common to all such affairs, and the

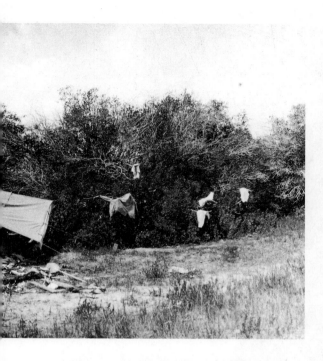

Nevills party set off to the cheers of the towns-people. So many famous river voyages began at that one little spot that it was later named Expedition Island and set aside as a National Historic Site (NHS) on November 24, 1968.

Below the town of Green River, the river flowed through mostly open country for about thirty miles. The first ten miles or so was prime bottomland, lined with willows and cotton-woods. The plentiful grass and easy availability of water meant that ranches were common, and many were established almost as soon as the railroad passed through. Well before the railroad came, though, ranchers and cattle-men recognized the value of the grazing lands along the Green. In 1849 a band of Cherokee Indians, displaced from their homeland east of the Mississippi River, decided to emigrate to

California and headed west with herds of cattle and horses. Reaching Browns Park late in the year, they wintered in that sheltered valley and resumed their journey the next spring. Their trail out of Browns Park came down Currant Creek, crossed the Green near the mouth of Black's Fork, and followed that stream to the mouth of its tributary, Ham's Fork.[3] The Church of Jesus Christ of Latter-day Saints (LDS) is reported to have grazed a herd of cattle in Browns Park in the 1850s. They prob-ably would have made their way through the Green River valley to get there, perhaps fol-lowing the same trail as the Cherokees.

Just below Green River City, in Cordwood Bottom, was the Harsha Ranch. In 1947 Norm Nevills sought shelter at the ranch from a mis-erable rain: "HARSHA RANCH. On right. Up to here we were suffering very acutely from the cold rain. Looking for a place to get shelter we spotted this ranch. Landing on right we wander back across a muddy field and discover a small, far from neat, children-filled house. But it's warm and out of the rain."[4] Not much is known about who established the ranch or when, near the head of the modern reservoir. Down-river a few miles was the Logan Ranch. In 1911 Ellsworth and Emery Kolb stopped there for their first night's camp on their photographic and film expedition from Wyoming to Mex-ico: "The Logan boys' ranch . . . was our first camp; but it will be one of the last to be for-gotten. The two Logan boys were sturdy, com-panionable young men, full of pranks, and of that bubbling, generous humor that flourishes

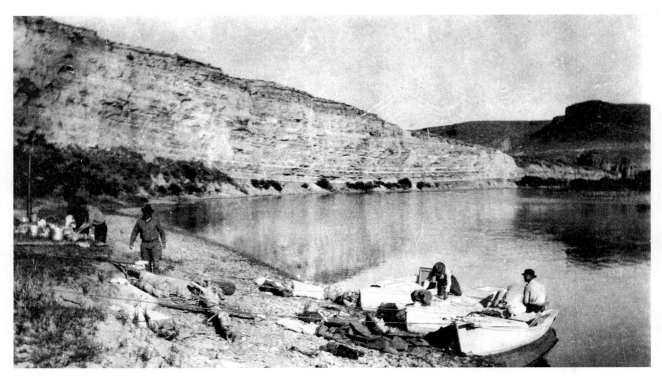

USGS party above Black's Fork, 1922.

in this Western Air."[5] The Logan brothers let the Kolbs use a storm cellar for a darkroom and told them to help themselves to the black-smith shop so they could make some alterations on their boats. By 1940, however, the ranch had fallen on hard times, as noted by Doris Nevills, who stopped there for lunch on June 20 of that year: "This is the filthiest place I have ever seen. Dogs, goats, and pigs all came down to the boats. A dirty woman with two small children comes down to talk. She tells us she caught the wildcat in the cage all by herself. How can people be so filthy when soap is so cheap?"[6] Norm agreed with her, noting in his diary "DO NOT STOP HERE IN FUTURE."

When he came down the Green again in 1947, he passed right by the ranch without a second thought.[7]

After the Logan Ranch, the landscape began to change. Badland buttes and spires appeared, and the river flowed through a low canyon. One of the members of the 1909 Galloway–Stone expedition left a detailed account of the river valley at this point:

The river continued in long bends through the rather narrow valley, terminating in low rocky barren hills tinted with all shades, from the gray lead colors through the yellow tints to a bright red. The stream

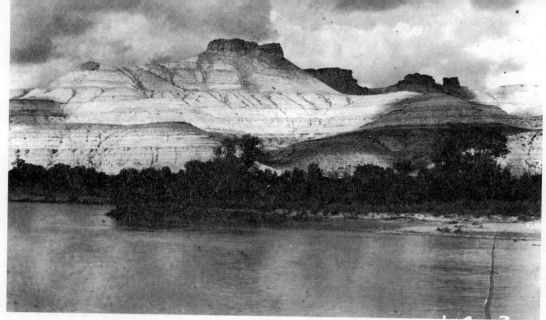
Firehole Towers, 1909.

washed a cliff on one side which turned the current across the valley in a series of bends until it struck the cliff on the other side, and then back again, and so on. The banks usually rose abruptly ten to twelve feet high which seemed to be about high water mark. The banks were usually lined with low willows not over ten feet high, also wild roses and in places with cotton-wood trees. Back of this the land was level for from a few feet—if water was not washing the face of a cliff—to a thousand feet or more. This low valley seemed to be the channel of the river at an earlier period when the flow was much greater in volume. It was thinly and irregularly covered with a stiff hard grass, which while not thorny was stiff enough to penetrate ordinary clothing. Here also was other forms of desert vegetation. The grass was near the water and very much in patches.[8]

Today the land along this stretch of river, down to the mouth of Black's Fork, is known as the Firehole Basin. The rocks on either side of the river are mostly part of Green River For-mation, a soft, easily eroded layer that forms buttes and chimneys and is common through-out southwestern Wyoming.[9] The area had little bottomland for grazing, usually only where side streams such as Potter Creek and Sage Creek entered the river and in the intrigu-ingly named Slippery Jim Bottom. Though this stretch was of little use to ranchers, who saw it as worthless badlands, others saw beauty in the shapes and colors. Cid Ricketts Sumner of the 1955 Hatch–Eggert Expedition described the surroundings:

Gradually the scene around us altered. The buttes on one side rose higher and more color came into them; red and buff mixed with the gray brown. Some were ribboned

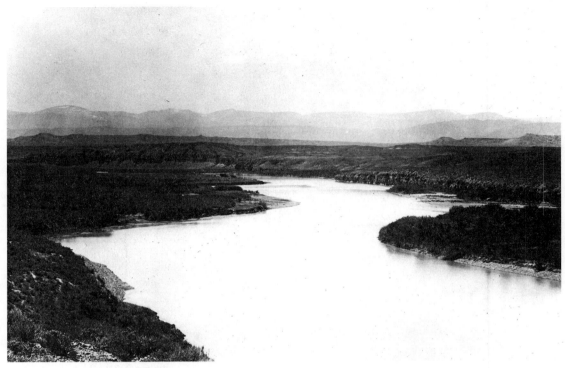

First view of the Uinta Mountains, just below Black's Fork.

masses topped now and then with a small nipple, reminding me of the Paps of Jura. At times these formations were close to the riverside, again they were set back beyond a level stretch of green woods and grasses or a bleak expanse of shale. Then, as the buttes grew higher, turreted castles appeared.[10]

A brochure advertising Reynolds-Hallacy River Expeditions down the Green in 1951 even mentioned the Firehole country as a selling point: "The unique trips, as organized, offer a variety of combinations, from one-day trips that voyage swiftly though smoothly through the striking colors and buttes of the three Firehole basins of the Green."[11]

At the mouth of Black's Fork, twenty-seven miles below Green River City, the landscape changed once again, opening back up, and river travelers got their first view of the distant Uinta Mountains, a seemingly impassable barrier. Even though they were some forty miles downriver, the lofty Uintas were never out of sight after this point. Just below the mouth of Black's Fork, at Currant Creek, was the Holmes Ranch, established by Walter and Emma Holmes around 1908. This was the best-known ranch along the river; it was a favored stop for anyone traveling down

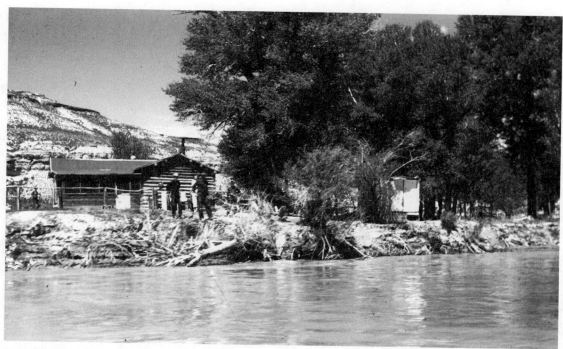

Holmes Ranch, 1952.

the Green from 1911, when the Kolb brothers stayed there, until Mrs. Holmes finally moved to Green River City in 1954. According to a neighbor, Lee Roy Brinegar, Walter Holmes was a "gentleman farmer," originally from England, who always wore a suit and tie and had only a few cows on his 190-acre ranch. He raised tumbling pigeons and fighting cocks at his ranch, while Emma Holmes kept a large vegetable garden and raised produce such as radishes, onions, and lettuce for sale in Green River.[12] Like many other ranchers along the river, they built a ferry to get back and forth across the river.

Just about every river traveler from 1909 on stopped at the ranch and commented on the fine hospitality afforded by Mr. and Mrs. Holmes; stories of evenings spent listening to tales of the Wild West in the Holmes ranch house are universal among river travelers down the upper Green for the first half of the twentieth century. This description comes from Ellsworth Kolb, who visited there in September 1911:

Our next camp was at the Holmes' ranch, a few miles below Black's Fork. We tried to buy some eggs of Walter Holmes, and were told that we could have them on one condition—that we visit him that evening. This was a price we were only too glad to pay, and the evening will linger long in

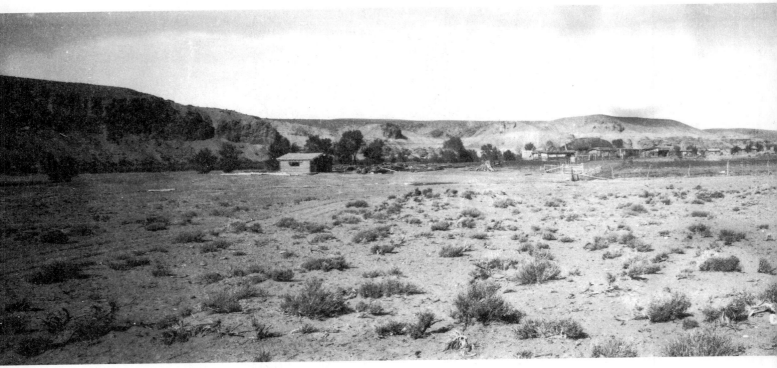

Holmes Ranch panorama, 1922.

our memories. Mr. Holmes entertained us with stories of hunting trips—after big game in the wilds of Colorado; and among the lakes of the Wind River Mountains, the distant source of the Green River. Mrs. Holmes and two young ladies entertained us with music; [and] it was late that night when we rolled ourselves in our blankets, on the banks twenty feet above the river.[13]

Antoine de Seynes, a French kayaker, passed by the ranch in 1938, along with Bernard de Colmont and Bernard's new bride, Geneviève, on one of the first kayak trips along the upper Green. All three of the French kayakers were much impressed by the cowboys of the Wild West:

The ranch was made up of a bunch of separate buildings, very simple and constructed in the manner of log cabins, horizontal tree trunks grouted with mud and a couple of corrals with thick log fences. Mr. Holmes who [*sic*] built everything, hauling the wood from some thirty miles away. He was the one who, in the middle of this desert, planted the few trees which surrounded the house, and he irrigates the few fields that he cultivates,

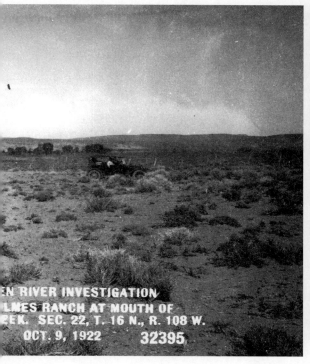

EN RIVER INVESTIGATION
LMES RANCH AT MOUTH OF
EK. SEC. 22, T. 16 N., R. 108 W.
OCT. 9, 1922   32395

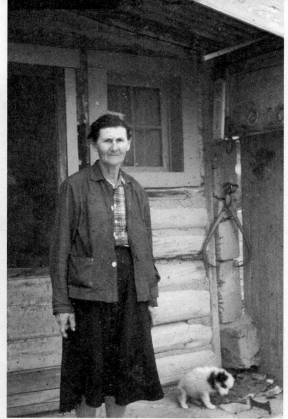

Emma Holmes.

where Mrs. Holmes is working at the moment [with] their two cowboys.[14]

Walter Holmes died in 1942, but Emma stayed at the ranch for most of the rest of her life.[15] Norman Nevills, a pioneer river outfitter, stopped at the Holmes Ranch twice, in 1940 and again in 1947. The first time the wind was howling and he stayed only briefly, noting that he got "canteen water here. Two elderly people who have seen and met all the river parties to date starting with Kolbs. Nice couple. Leave here with awfully hard upstream wind."[16] In 1947 his party spent more time there, enjoying the company of the widow Holmes:

HOLMES RANCH. Stopped here in '40. Mrs. Holmes takes a keen interest in all the river parties. Mr. Holmes has died since we were here last, but Mrs. Holmes carries on alone, with occasional help from nephews etc. We bring in our lunch. All ride a horse, principally Joan. Generally enjoy ourselves loafing around.[17]

The next day Mrs. Holmes showed them an "ancient" Ford Model T, which they were able to start, so Otis Marston, one of the Nevills boatmen, could catch the stage back to Green River to look for his camera at the Harsha Ranch (he had actually left it in the station wagon at Green River, when they were launching the boats). Maradel Marston, who was on the same 1947 trip, was very impressed by Emma Holmes: "Mrs. Holmes is a remarkable woman of about 70 who runs the ranch completely by herself. She is tall and very capably strong. She grows her own food. Her hair is brown and she has large blue fascinating eyes."[18]

But sometimes hospitality brought obligations. In a 1952 letter to Phil Lundstrom, Otis Marston described a boating party who stopped at the ranch to enjoy Emma Holmes's generosity but felt obliged to return a favor: "I suppose Garth told you that Holmes died but, at latest reports, Mrs. Holmes is still running the ranch. The last boat party thru there stopped and Mrs. Holmes was troubled with a cow that had died in a shed. The two lads of the party had to cut the carcass up and take it out for her. It cost them their breakfasts."[19]

By the 1950s Emma Holmes was an institution along the upper Green. An article in the local *Green River Star* described a trip:

down to Holmes' ferry at Buckboard Sunday to pick up AK [Reynolds, son of the owner of the newspaper] and Lug and a group from Rock Springs who had run the Firehole in AK's boats that day . . . briefly saw that grand personage, Emma Holmes, who had come across the river on a chair, pulling along a cable hand over hand . . . bringing Pete and Mary Ewen . . . who had been down to lend a hand at the Holmes place over the weekend . . . Mrs. Holmes was in a hurry . . . she has no help at the ranch right now and had all the evening's chores to do . . . that lady is one to be long remembered . . . haying, irrigating, riding for cattle . . . doing whatever becomes necessary to keep the ranch on an even keel and functioning . . . she is of the real stuff that has made the women of the West such grand people . . . and who have made the West a grand place to live.[20]

A few miles below the Holmes Ranch, in Halfway Hollow, was the Buckboard Hotel, a small hostelry established to serve travelers on the route between the little towns of Manila and Linwood, Utah, and Green River, Wyoming. By wagon or horseback, it was about a two-day journey from Linwood or Manila to Green River, and the hotel was situated at the halfway point. William Purdy, the principal of the school in Manila, Utah, noted in a salvage report: "Peter Wall noticed that people traveling from one settlement to the other had to camp out one night. He decided to relieve their discomforts, and make a good investment besides, by building the hotel on the banks of the Green in 1912." Wall was described variously as a "go-getter, a good talker," and a "smart politician."[21] He also ran a freight line between Manila and Green River and therefore thought that the hotel was a good idea. But cars and trucks had arrived and roads had improved by the time he built it, so the hotel sat mostly empty, visited only by the curious and

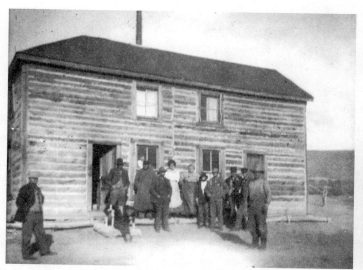
Buckboard Hotel. *Courtesy Sweetwater County Museum.*

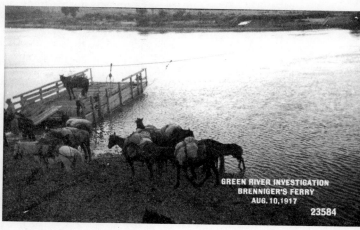
GREEN RIVER INVESTIGATION
BRENNIGER'S FERRY
AUG. 10, 1917
23584

Brinegar's Ferry.

local teenagers. It was the site of some merriment, however, and was used occasionally for dances and other local events. Barbara Williams Amburn, who grew up on a ranch on Henry's Fork, said that people would gather there for dances in the 1950s, including a Halloween dance in which the old hotel was made into a spook alley and everyone dressed in costume. It was finally torn down while the dam was being built.[22] A ranch by the same name was also located there, as well as a ford across the river, which was the site of a fine swimming hole.

Below Halfway Hollow were more ranches, such as the John Lowe Ranch on Bridger Bottoms. Ralf Woolley, a USGS surveyor, noted in 1922 that the family "came out to greet us and bade us God speed on our journey."[23] Next downriver was the Brinegar Ranch, established by William Brinegar and his wife,

Maddie, sometime before 1917. William and a ranch hand built the three-bedroom log cabin. They ran sheep on the hills on both sides of the river, so they built a ferry. It had several iterations: the first was too small, and the next one washed away in a flood. So Brinegar had a heavy-duty ferry built in Green River and floated down the river to the crossing. The ferry, attached to a cable, used the pressure of the current to push it back and forth across the river. A wagon wheel could be used to turn the ferry's nose into the current. If the water was low, they had to push it across with poles—no easy task with up to a hundred sheep on board! The Brinegars kept a few cows for milk and meat and grew alfalfa for their sheep, even though the irrigation made the mosquito problem worse.[24]

The sluggish river made this stretch a heaven for mosquitoes and a hell for animals and people alike. The river slowed and widened, meandering across open bottomlands that provided excellent grazing but were also home to clouds of mosquitoes that feasted on anyone unfortunate enough to be there during the hatch. Mosquitoes had no doubt plagued the Indians and were a trial for travelers from the earliest days. Warren Angus Ferris, who came west with a party of trappers in 1830, wrote: "[W]e were nearly victimized by moschetoes [*sic*], which during the five days of our vicinity to this stream [the Green River], kept sucking at the vital currents in our veins in spite of every precaution that could be taken."[25] Writing in 1922, USGS surveyor Ralf Woolley noted a "battle royal" with the stinging pests:

> After supper the camp was invaded by swarms of mosquitoes. Smudges were kindled but they were only partially effective; the mosquitoes were apparently too hungry to be cheated out of a good meal by a little smoke so we had a battle royal, not only during the evening but all night long. The result was that in the morning all felt like they had had a pretty rough night.[26]

Mary Beckwith, a passenger on a Mexican Hat Expeditions river trip in June 1956, the worst time of the year, wrote: "Looking back upstream we are convulsed with laughter. Each boat is animated with flying arms, shirts and what-have-you in annihilation of the pests. Could we be termed a 'mosquito fleet'?"[27]

Sandbars were also a problem for river runners in the days before the dam; the river, meandering through its open valley, was shallow except at the flood in May and June. Many early river runners preferred to travel later in the year, when the water had gone down, and were constantly pulling their boats over gravel and sandbars. "Many sand-bars kept us guessing as to where the deepest channel of the stream was, and sometimes poor guesses hung the boats up on bars," noted Ralf Woolley in 1922.[28] Sandbars were good crossing places for cattle and horses, but river runners cursed them.

This stretch was not an easy place to make a ranch successful, despite the pasturelike river bottoms and free grass. Ralf Woolley noted in 1922 that some of the ranches they passed were "abandoned, and at the others the occupants were fighting a desperate battle with alkali and other obstacles in an effort to make a home."[29] Not far below the Kraus Ranch, opposite the mouth of Marsh Creek about fifty miles below Green River City, the river cut through the first of a series of hogbacks formed along the flanks of the rising Uinta Mountains. Once past the first ridge, the river reentered open country for another few miles, passing the mouth of Henry's Fork.

This location had long been a favorite camping spot of the Shoshones; it provided good water and grazing for their horses, fish in the river, and shade from the cottonwoods. The mosquitoes could be fearsome in certain seasons, but their numbers diminished later in the summer. Some of the old mountain men chose the lush bottomlands around Henry's Fork as a place to settle (as noted above), and the area had ranches from the late 1800s on. It was at the mouth of Henry's Fork that Ashley planned to have the first rendezvous, even though he later moved it up Henry's Fork to Burnt Fork, Utah, about twenty miles up Henry's Fork (see chapter 1). He was not the only river traveler to make a cache at the mouth of Henry's Fork; in 1869 John Wesley Powell buried a supply of rations and extra scientific instruments there. When he learned that a party of Indians had been camping in the area for some weeks, he was afraid that the cache might have been discovered and raided but was relieved to find it undisturbed: "Our fears are soon allayed, for we find it all right. Our chronometer wheels are not taken for hair ornaments; our barometer tubes, for beads; nor the sextant thrown into the river as 'bad medicine,' as had been predicted."[30]

Naturally, with lush grass and good water, the mouth of Henry's Fork was a favorite place for cattle. In addition to the retired mountain men, some of the earliest small cattle ranchers along the river got their start there. Judge William A. Carter, the sutler at Fort Bridger and a famous figure in Wyoming history, grazed large herds of cattle around Henry's Fork in the 1870s. As was common in the west, unbranded cattle were considered fair game. A historian has written: "To this day, there is a saying on Henry's Fork that all of the local ranches were started with Judge Carter's cattle."[31] One

of those taking advantage of the Judge's herds was Elijah "Lije" Driscoll, who first came to Fort Bridger with Col. Patrick Connor's California Volunteers during the Civil War. Driscoll stayed on after the war and started a ranch near the mouth of Henry's Fork in 1868, along with his Shoshone wife. His herds expanded rapidly, and he took advantage of the coming of the railroad to trade cattle. Shadrach "Shade" Large settled on a ranch near the line that separated Wyoming from Utah territory shortly afterward and later moved into Uncle Jack Robinson's old cabin. Large, married to a Shoshone woman who was reportedly a granddaughter of Sacajawea, was said to be a rough character; he lived around the Green River until he died as a result of a fall from his horse in 1897.[32]

In the early years of the twentieth century Peter Finch ran a small ranch at the mouth of Henry's Fork. But the bottomlands around the mouth of Henry's Fork were not really developed until 1930, when the Williams family bought Finch out and settled there. That year Henry Williams, the patriarch of this energetic family, left the mines in Atlantic City, Wyoming, borrowed money from his brother, and started a new life on Henry's Fork with his wife, Maude; their four sons Henry, Bill, Jared, and Paul; and five daughters. Together they bought 1,200 acres at the mouth of Henry's Fork, including the old Finch place, Dewey Lamb's small ranch, the Driscoll Ranch, and another small ranch owned by the Hereford family. They also owned land across the river and up

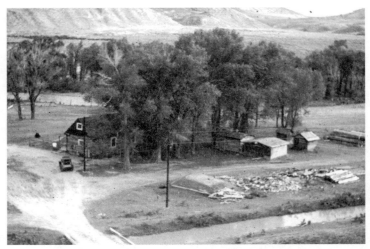
Williams Ranch on Henry's Fork. *Courtesy Barbara Williams Amburn.*

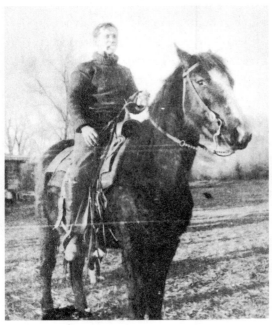
Keith Smith.

on Little Mountain and Goslin Mountain in Wyoming, where they grazed their herds in the summer. The Williams brothers built houses, corrals, fences, and outbuildings, put up hay grown in the lush meadows, developed springs, dug ditches, and made many other improvements on the main ranch on Henry's Fork and also built cow camps, wild horse corrals, and sheep dip tanks elsewhere on their property.

One of the Williams daughters, Mabel, became a county nurse and later married a local man named Nels Philbrick, who was likewise busy. Nels had a gas station in Manila and started his own electric company to bring power to the remote town. He also built his own flat-bottomed boat powered by an aircraft engine and propeller, which he called the "Flying Dutchman." The Williams family prospered in their ranch on Henry's Fork until the construction of Flaming Gorge Dam inundated their property.[33]

Just a few miles up Henry's Fork was the little town of Linwood.[34] The site was purchased by George Solomon in the late 1890s, during the Lucerne Valley land boom. Like many such companies at the time, the Lucerne Land and Water Company promised more irrigation water than it could deliver, and Solomon soon grew discouraged. He sold his interest to the family of Keith Smith, a well-educated (Andover and Yale) and ambitious young man from back East. When the Smiths suffered some economic reverses in Massachusetts, Keith and his brother Sanford settled on cattle ranching as a way to repair the family fortunes and came west to look for a suitable place to start a ranch. While traveling through eastern Utah, Smith heard about the possibilities of the Lucerne Valley and the Green River country. An inspection of the lands north of the Uinta Mountains convinced him that this was the place. In the summer of 1902 Keith and his father, who was a "complete tenderfoot," arrived in Green River, Wyoming. There they were greeted by Sanford and Ole Neilson, a local homesteader they had met earlier that year in Vernal, Utah. Sanford and Ole had built a sixteen-foot boat at Green River, into which they loaded "$500 worth of ranch supplies including a ton of wire fencing," purchased at Montgomery Ward in Chicago.[35] With Sanford at the tiller, Keith and Ole ("a giant of a man") using two-by-four boards as oars, and Keith's father sitting in the back, they set off. Amazingly, despite being "unwieldy," this craft made it all the way down the Green to Ole's ranch at Neilson's Flat in four days.

Smith and his family eventually settled on a place a few miles above the mouth of Henry's Fork and set to work. Within a year of his arrival he and his brother had cleared acres of sagebrush and built a ranch house, outbuildings, corrals and fences, and even two bridges: one across the Green, sturdy enough for cattle, horses, and people, and one across Henry's Fork that could hold cars and trucks.[36] Smith later purchased a couple of run-down ranches to expand his operations and brought energy and skills that seldom had been seen in the remote valley of the Green River.[37]

Next the members of this busy family turned their sights on developing the town of Linwood.[38] In the first decades of the twentieth century Linwood was a thriving small community, serving the many ranches and farms in the area. At one time Linwood had a school, built right on the Utah-Wyoming line, so that part of it was in each state. It was the only school to be served by two different state school boards. The town also had a gas station, an octagonal dance hall called the Roundhouse, which boasted a finely polished wood floor, a number of homes, and the Smith and Larsen Mercantile Company, run by Keith's father. The site had featured a post office since 1893. Keith moved it from the Wyoming side of town to a room in his store and took over as postmaster in 1906.[39] The little hamlet served as a supply point for the many ranches in the area. After sheep were introduced, Linwood's population grew several-fold during the shearing season.[40] That season tended to bring a more lawless element, and the town saw its share of the Wild West. One resident of nearby Browns Park, Charlie Crouse, sometimes passed through Linwood on his way back to his remote ranch. His sons, Clarence and Stanley, found other ways to attract notice in Linwood:

Crouse's children themselves were a bit wild. In one instance his two sons, Clarence and Stanley, drunk, rode into Linwood, Utah, stark naked, roped a local blacksmith and part-time deputy sheriff and craps dealer, Pete Miller, and dragged Miller around town. Ultimately, two locals rescued Miller. Miller was employed at a gambling establishment and saloon just

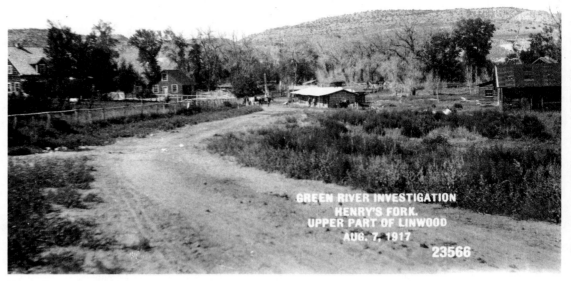

Linwood, 1917.

across the border in Wyoming, known as the "Bucket of Blood."[41]

The Bucket of Blood, built and operated by Bob Swift at the end of the 1800s, was notorious for "liquor, gambling, and 'questionable' women." Like most of Linwood, it was built close to the state line, which gave it an advantage for anyone who got too rowdy or was on the lookout for the sheriff. They could "elude the law by changing jurisdictions. All that was necessary was to step out the back door."[42] Many who frequented the Bucket of Blood made sure to keep an eye on the door. The remote canyons of the upper Green were a good place to avoid being seen, and outlaws who were said to have spent time in Linwood

included Butch Cassidy, the Sundance Kid, Matt Warner, Elzy Lay, and Isom Dart, among many others. Even Jesse and Frank James reportedly spent a winter hiding out nearby, coming to the Bucket of Blood for company and entertainment. The Bucket of Blood finally burned down in the early twentieth century and was never rebuilt.

Linwood was also the downstream terminus of the proposed Green River Navigation Company, established in March 1908 by a group of Green River and Rock Springs business leaders. The idea was to build a steamboat to carry passengers and freight from the railroad at Green River down to the ranches around Linwood, thus avoiding the two-day trip over rough roads between the two towns.

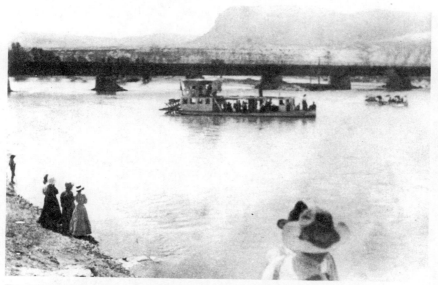

The steamboat *Comet*'s maiden voyage, 1908. *Courtesy Wyoming State Archives, Department of State Parks and Cultural Resources.*

After boilers and a steam engine were obtained from Chicago, the steamboat was built in Green River and christened the *Comet*. The $25,000, 60-foot long craft was launched on July 4, 1908, with the maiden voyage scheduled for July 7. Passengers included the officers of the Green River Navigation Company and local dignitaries, refreshed by "ample supplies of beer." Linwood was reached after a journey of only eight hours, far quicker than the two days it took to reach it overland. The return voyage, however, was not so easy. It took thirty-three hours to make the same journey against the current, and the deep draft of the *Comet* proved to be unsuitable for the shallow Green. It frequently had to be hauled off sandbars with winches and finally ran out of coal. A second voyage, hauling freight for Linwood,

proved to be no more successful, and after that the trip to Linwood was not tried again. Today only the bell of the *Comet* survives, in the Green River Rotary Club. Two other vessels, the *Sunbeam* and the patriotically named *Teddy R*, were no more successful.[43]

Below Henry's Fork was only a short stretch of open country before the river entered Flaming Gorge, known locally as Ashley's Flat; at low water it had a shallow ford known as Ashley's Crossing.[44] In these last few slow miles, the Green remained wide and wandering, as if reluctant to enter the constricted canyons below. But after gathering itself at the head of Flaming Gorge, it plunged into the shadows. For the next forty miles, all the way to Browns Park, with only a few exceptions, the river would be confined by deep canyons.

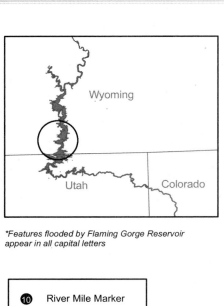

Wyoming

Utah   Colorado

*Features flooded by Flaming Gorge Reservoir
appear in all capital letters*

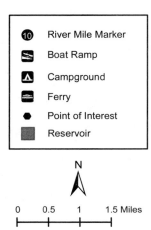

⑩	River Mile Marker
⛴	Boat Ramp
⛺	Campground
⛴	Ferry
●	Point of Interest
▨	Reservoir

N

0   0.5   1   1.5 Miles

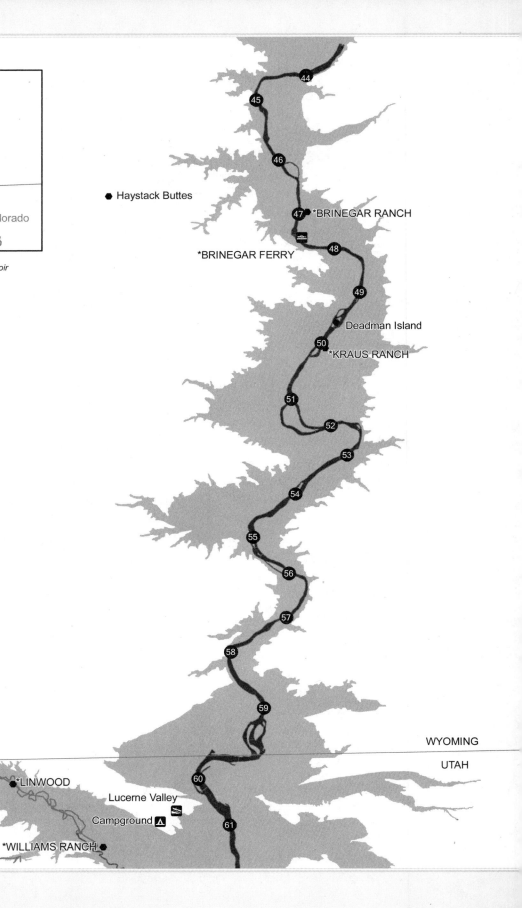

● Haystack Buttes

44

45

46

47 ●*BRINEGAR RANCH

*BRINEGAR FERRY

48

49

Deadman Island

50 *KRAUS RANCH

51

52

53

54

55

56

57

58

59

WYOMING

UTAH

60

●*LINWOOD

Henry's Fork

Lucerne Valley

Campground ⛺

61

*WILLIAMS RANCH ●

CANYONS AND RAPIDS

The bright July sun sparkled on the almost unruffled surface of the river. Our last bits of contact with civilization—the Forest Service campground known as Hideout, and a gradually settling pall of dust from our departing vehicles— vanished from sight upstream. Silently we drifted into the beautiful canyon wilderness of the upper Green River, accessible only by boat ... Were it not for the fact that the shoreline seemed to move by at a rapid rate, we might have felt as though we were suspended in timeless, motionless space, so quiet had been the river ... Great ledges of red sandstone receded in steps, towering several thousand feet above the canyon floor. A lush growth of spruce, ponderosa pine, and mountain juniper covered the walls. Here and there aspens shimmered in the sunlight, yellow-green patches of brilliant contrast. We sighted deer along the shore and we were constantly startling wild geese ... The river, far from its source in the Wind River mountains, was large and murky, paced with latent power ...

The Green did the work while we lazily drifted along, enthralled by the untouched beauty about us. The river began to drop in easy steps, each a long pool, quiet and glassy, leading to a slick tongue of faster water where we always had the sensation of a sudden drop in river elevation. The tongue would invariably break up into a rash of waves, exciting but not dangerous.

—"FOLBOTS THROUGH DINOSAUR" (1952)

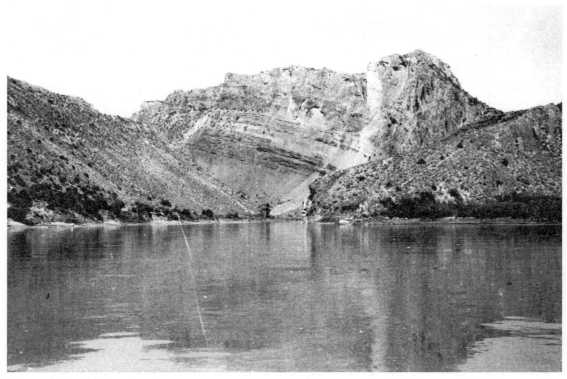

Entrance to Flaming Gorge.

Flaming Gorge

The entrances and exits of rivers from mountain ranges are often scenic and even dramatic, but few are more spectacular than Flaming Gorge, the place where the Green River enters the Uinta Mountains. Even today, when the lower portion is covered by the still waters of the reservoir, it excites admiration and draws attention. The story of how the Green cut its canyon down the spine of the Uinta Mountains is better told by geologists. Briefly, when the Uintas began to rise during the Laramide Orogeny some 60 million years ago, the forces created faulting and folding. This resulted in hogback ridges paralleling the east-west trend of the mountains. One of these, the Boars Tusk, towers more than 1,500 feet over the site of Linwood and the mouth of Henry's Fork. The Green River cut through these hogbacks and into the very heart of the mountains in a process still not fully understood and well outside the scope of this book. In doing so, it cut through various layers that had been tilted up by the faulting, resulting in dramatic changes in geology in short distances. Flaming Gorge itself gets its brilliant red color from the Moenkopi and Chinle Formations, while Horseshoe Canyon cuts through the Park City Formation and Phosphoria Formation, which has been extensively mined for phosphates to the south, near Vernal, Utah. Kingfisher Canyon brings the cliffs of Weber Sandstone to the surface. Finally, in Red Canyon, the river has cut through the deep red Uinta Mountain Quartzite, the oldest and hardest rocks in the region. No wonder it takes a trained geologist to make any kind of sense out of this jumble of rocks, no fewer than "33 exposed formations that regionally add up to nearly 72,000 vertical feet—almost 14 miles—of rock, spanning as much as 3 billion years of geologic history. Within that 3-billion-year span, 14 known unconformities represent about 2 billion years of missing rocks."[1]

While geologists might debate the effects of compressional deformation and stream capture, the effect that this remarkable landscape had on river travelers who viewed these scenes from the river or from overland is beyond dispute. It was here that river travelers first saw the aptly named Flaming Gorge, where the river entered the Uintas through a narrow cleft in towering red cliffs over 1,000 feet higher than the river. From upriver, it appeared that the river was flowing into a cave in the mountains, giving some early explorers anxious moments. The alarm felt by William Manly as he floated the Green on his way to California in 1849 has already been noted, but he was not alone in remarking on the scene just below Linwood, as the river came up against the flanks of the Uintas. In 1886 F. E. Shearer wrote: "At the mouth of Henry's Fork there is a view on Green River of great beauty, which derives its principal charm from its vivid colors. The waters of the river are of the purest emerald, with banks and sand-bars of glistening white. The perpendicular bluff to the left is nearly 1,500 feet above the level of the river, and of a bright red and yellow. When illuminated by full sunlight, it is grand, and deserves its full title 'The Flaming Gorge.'"[2] Ralf Woolley, the USGS engineer in charge of the 1922 damsite survey, abandoned his usual dispassionate style and waxed eloquent about the canyon: "[T]he north wall of Flaming Gorge, with its vivid hues of red, brown, and ocher, rises like a huge flame of fire ahead. The gorge . . . forms a very impressive entrance to the series of canyons below."[3] Frederick S. Dellenbaugh, who accompanied John Wesley Powell's second expedition in 1871, was the first to see beyond the mythical "Green River Suck" to the beauty of the canyon:

> Just below the mouth of Henry's Fork [the river] doubled to the left and we found ourselves between two low cliffs, then in a moment we dashed to the right into the beautiful canyon, whose summit we had seen, rising about 1300 feet on the right, and a steep slope on the left at the base of which was a small bottom covered with

all cottonwood trees, whose green shone resplendent against the red rocks. . . . The canyon was surprisingly beautiful and romantic.[4]

The Green River Suck

The mythical but nonetheless dreaded Green River Suck was supposed to be a deadly cataract somewhere on the Green River that was impossible to pass safely; even attempting it was to court a certain death in its roiling, dangerous waters. During high-water periods, the water pooled and swirled as it entered Flaming Gorge. The resulting whirlpools gave rise to the legend of the Suck.[5] The story began during the Ashley Days of the fur trappers, and it's impossible to say just who first told the tale around a campfire. It first appeared in print in 1856, in the memoirs of James P. Beckwourth, an African American trapper who styled himself the "Chief of the Crow Nation." Beckwourth, a former slave, was in Ashley's party that came across the plains in 1825. In his memoirs, narrated to an admiring and credulous writer in a California gold camp in the 1850s, Beckwourth claimed to have rescued Ashley from the Green River Suck when Ashley fell out of their buffalo-skin boat: "The current . . . became exceedingly rapid, and drew towards the centre from each shore. This place we named the Suck. This fall continued for six or eight miles, making a sheer descent, in the entire distance, of upwards of two hundred and fifty feet."[6] Beckwourth goes on to relate in breathless prose how he swam to Ashley, who held onto his shoulders, and started to swim for shore. But the current was too strong, and soon they were in danger of being dragged to "inevitable death." Just when Beckwourth's strength was giving out, Thomas Fitzpatrick reached out a pole and pulled Beckwourth to safety, with Ashley still clinging to his shoulders.[7]

This all makes a great story, except that it was sheer fabrication. Neither Beckwourth nor Fitzpatrick was with Ashley on the river. Beckwourth was in the Wind River Mountains, far to the north, with James Clyman, while Fitzpatrick was exploring the northern slopes of the Uintas. But the legend took hold and grew, even as its location moved. The Suck was variously placed at Ashley Falls, Disaster Falls in the Canyon of Lodore, Split Mountain Canyon (where Ashley actually did fall out of the boat, although he was quickly rescued by two unnamed men), and a number of other locales. As the location shifted, so did the results; in some versions all save Ashley himself or Ashley and one other companion were drowned. In others they survived but lost all their boats and equipment and were forced to wander across the sagebrush plains until rescued by Indians. Some stories even had them resorting to cannibalism! It mattered little to the mountain men that none of these events actually occurred. The ability to tell a good lie was as highly valued as skill at setting traps or skinning a beaver. In reality, once the river made it into the canyon it sorted itself out quickly and flowed with hardly a ripple until it entered Red Canyon.

Even though none of Beckwourth's story is true, it still conveys a good idea of the imagined dangers that lurked in the remote canyons of the Green. There was indeed fast water there. Barbara Williams Amburn remembers that whenever they moved cattle to their pastures on the other side of the river they had to go a considerable distance upriver from the mouth of Henry's Fork before pushing the herd into the river to swim across, because of the turbulent water above the entrance to Flaming Gorge. But it was not the dark portal of doom that the stories made it out to be. The dread of the Suck and other supposed dangers in the canyons of the Green was strongest in Green River but held less sway closer to the canyons. When Ellsworth and Emery Kolb were getting ready to start their river voyage in Green River in September 1911, they were told over and over that they would never make it, that the Suck would drag them to inevitable doom. As they traveled downriver and stopped at the ranches along the way, however, they were surprised and somewhat reassured to note that "there were comments by some of the men on our venture, but they lacked the true Green River tang. Here, close to the upper canyons, the unreasonable fear of the rapids gave way to a reasonable respect for them."[8]

Horseshoe Canyon

Less than two miles below the dramatic entrance at Flaming Gorge, the river made a long U-shaped bend known as Horseshoe Canyon. Horseshoe Canyon was spectacular

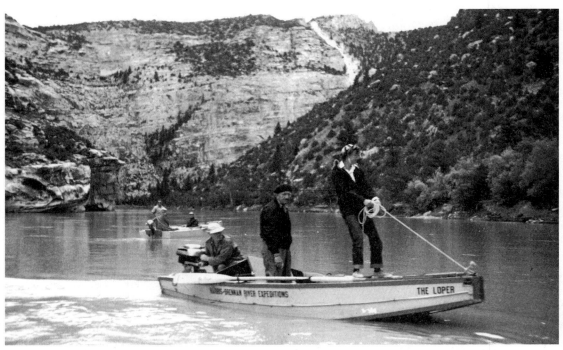

Horseshoe Canyon.

evidence of the dramatic geological forces that had accompanied the creation of the Uintas. Like Flaming Gorge, Horseshoe was a short canyon, only three miles long; but unlike the flaring red rocks of Flaming Gorge, Horseshoe was composed of gray limestone and shale. The change of color and mood of the canyons was abrupt.

On his solo voyage down the river in October 1937, Buzz Holmstrom found the two canyons delightful: "Horseshoe and King-fisher Canyons, short and rapid-free, filled with sunshine and the songs of countless birds and the call of geese and ducks high overheard broken only by the intermit-tent splash of jumping fish. The tree-lined

shores interspersed with deer and beavers surely made this the answer to a sportsman's prayers."[9]

Horseshoe Canyon was not totally free of rapids, however; it had a small riffle (minor rapid) at the apex of the U shape, caused by rocks washed in by a small, steep side canyon. In his 1871 report John Wesley Powell made much of this:

Now the river turns abruptly around a point to the right, and the waters plunge swiftly down among great rocks; and here we have our first experience with can-yon rapids. I stand up on the deck of my boat to seek a way among the wave

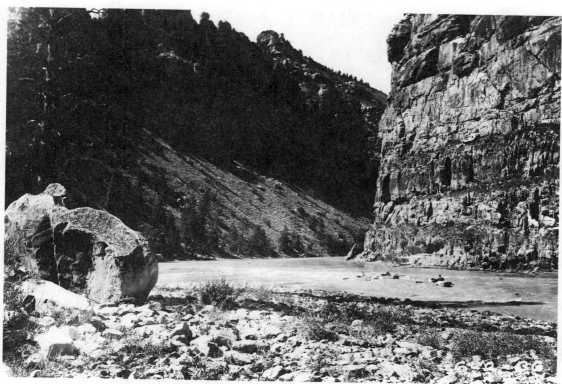
Rapid at the turn of Horseshoe Canyon.

beaten rocks. All untried as we are with such waters, the moments are filled with intense anxiety. Soon our boats reach the swift current; a stroke or two, now on this side, now on that, and we thread the narrow passage with exhilarating velocity, mounting the high waves, whose foaming crests dash over us, and plunging into the troughs, until we reach the quiet water below; and then comes a feeling of great relief. Our first rapid is run.[10]

Powell's breathless description of the "wave beaten rocks" caused much derision among later river travelers, for his description was about as accurate as the tales of the Green River Suck. A rapid can loom larger than it really is when run for the first time, but this is a good example of Powell's tendency toward hyperbole. If later river runners mention the little riffle at all, they usually dismiss it as Otis Marston did in his notes on his 1947 trip with Norm Nevills, calling it "small and docile."[11] Nevills himself noted that the rapid was "leveled over by the high water," the same time of year when Powell came down. Nevills went on to say: "We are all terribly impressed by the unusual beauty of this, Horseshoe

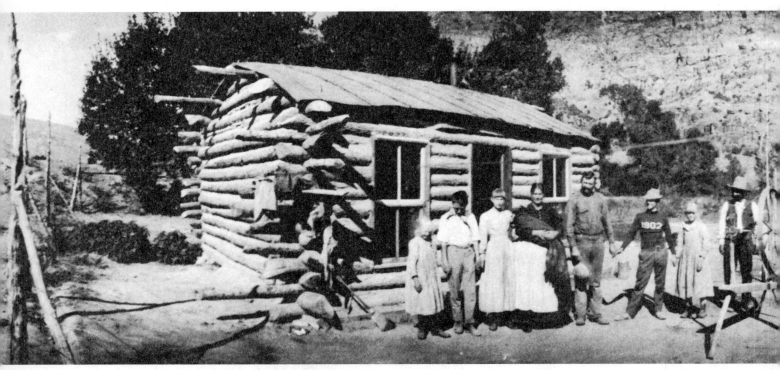

Ole Nielson's cabin, Nielson's Flat, 1902.

Canyon. Not alone is the change so great from the barren canyons above here, but this canyon is outstanding."[12] Mary Beckwith, on a 1956 Mexican Hat Expeditions trip, was equally blasé about Powell's first rapid: "On we glide, past Powell's 'little gem of a rapid'—their first and a big thrill. To us—a ruffle around a rock."[13]

Neilson's Flat

Below Horseshoe Canyon the river entered an open area called Neilson's Flat, named for Ole Neilson, who had settled there with his wife around 1900. The Neilsons put a lot of work into their ranch, which was accessible only by river or by a road that came down Sheep Creek. They were helped by their good friend Keith Smith, later of Linwood. In the summer of 1902 Smith, his brother Sanford, his father, and Ole Neilson brought a cumbersome boat down the river, loaded with supplies so that the Smiths could establish a ranch:

This is where we spent the summer... We ate our meals in their cabin. Ole taught me to harness a team and I helped him to build a barbed wire fence around his garden. Also we put up hay six miles up Sheep Creek... Father was uncomplaining in a life utterly new to him. He and I used to fish a good deal in Sheep Creek, and on an outdoor table we played dominoes, one of which was taken by Mrs. Neilson's pet magpie. When the magpie died, Mrs. Neilson thought that Father had killed it. Our trunk was housed in the cabin, and in it I kept the letters I received and a prized box of Bock Panatella cigars. The latter gradually disappeared. When we came upon Mrs. Neilson smoking one of our prized Panatellas one day, she explained that her baby, whom she called Little Cuss, had helped himself to a cigar and sucked it. She said she was obliged to smoke it so that it would not be wasted.[14]

Ole Neilson was one of the stalwarts of the tiny community of Linwood but was killed in a boiler explosion at a sawmill in 1922.[15] After that his ranch fell on hard times, as noted by Ralf Woolley that same year:

Considerable work was done on Neilson's Flat at one time in an effort to make a ranch of it. There is a rather pretentious dwelling house, a barn, sheds, underground cellar, and a windlass device for raising water from the river in barrels for irrigation purposes. The place was deserted at the time of our visit, and looked as though it had not been occupied for a considerable time.[16]

In 1940 Norm Nevills stopped at Neilson's Flat to talk to a young couple from Denver who were irrigating a potato field with a small pump.[17] But by then any dreams of making a living in the remote area had all but vanished.

Kingfisher Canyon

As Powell passed through this canyon in 1869, he saw numerous examples of the belted kingfisher (*Megaceryle alcyon*), a medium-sized bird that lives along riverbanks, catching fish and other small animals.[18] They were so common in the stretch below Neilson's Flat that Powell decided to name the canyon after them: "Kingfishers are playing about the streams, and so we adopt as names Kingfisher Creek, Kingfisher Park, and Kingfisher Canyon."[19] In the short but spectacular Kingfisher Canyon, barely a mile in length, the geology changes once again, to tall cliffs of buff-colored Weber Sandstone, the same formation seen in Dinosaur National Monument's Echo Park area. Despite its charms, Kingfisher Canyon could be hazardous, as proven by Bus Hatch on his first river voyage in 1931. Hatch, still a novice boatman but always in charge of whatever he did, was at the oars, with his cousin, Frank Swain; his brother Tom; and his brother-in-law, Cap Mowrey, in the boat. Swain later reported: "We start at the head of Kingfisher Canyon. Hear rapid at bottom and I call out 'cataract ahead.' There is one rock in the middle with 40 acres on each side. Bus got excited and ended up on the rock and stove big hole in boat. Mowrey grabs tin and puts it over hole. Bus got within 12 feet from shore when boat sinks and we swim out."[20] The hole, as Cap

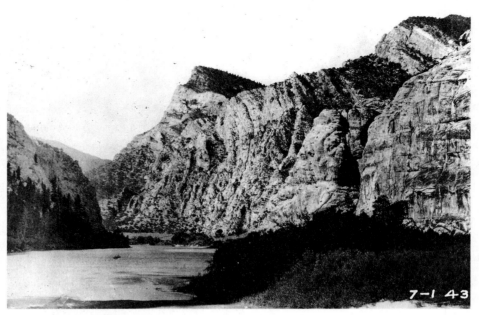

Mouth of Sheep Creek Canyon.

Mowrey later said, was "big enough to throw a cat through."[21] But Mowrey's quick thinking with the pie tin kept them from sinking in the middle of the channel. Fortunately, Bus, being a contractor, had brought along extra wood and tools, and a bucket of tar. They made repairs on the boat and continued their trip.

Powell's Kingfisher Creek is today set aside as Sheep Creek Canyon Geological Area by the U.S. Forest Service, due to its intriguing geology. Before the reservoir, a road down the canyon provided access to the river. River runners would often start their trips there to avoid the flat water, wind, and mosquitoes in the open country above. The road continued down the right (south) side of the river all the way to Hideout Flat. Sheep Creek was usually a clear and sparkling stream of good water, but it would run a flood of thick red mud whenever there was a big storm, due to the steepness of its canyon.[22] Despite its charms and the ease of access to the river, a number of early river runners reported swarms of mosquitoes in the river bottom around the mouth of Sheep Creek Canyon and hurried on. Just below was a footbridge built by the Civilian Conservation Corps (CCC) in the 1930s, which allowed sheep herders to get their herds across the river without resorting to a ferry.[23]

Hideout Flat

Beehive Point, at the end of Kingfisher Canyon, is further proof of how observant of bird life John Wesley Powell was. Beehive Point is a folded outcropping of Weber Sandstone, further evidence of the intense faulting that this whole area has undergone. It provided a home for thousands of swallows:

> Our general course this day has been south, but here the river turns to the east around a point which is rounded to the shape of a dome, and on its sides little cells have been carved by the action of the water; and in these pits, which cover the face of the dome, hundreds of swallows have built their nests. As they flit about the cliffs, they look like swarms of bees, giving to the whole the appearance of a colossal beehive of the old time form, and so we name it Beehive Point.[24]

There was also a small rapid at Beehive Point, another taste of things soon to come in Red Canyon. Below Beehive Point was a small open area known as Hideout Flat, the haunt of many outlaws who passed through the area during the heyday of the Wild Bunch. A hidden trail came down Hideout Draw, crossed at a secret ford there, and continued on the other side of the river. It was one of many such trails in eastern Utah used by people who wished to travel without notice. In 1911 the Kolb brothers encountered some suspicious characters not far from this part of the river:

> We had previously been informed that some of these mountains were the hiding -places of men who were "wanted" in the three states which bordered near here. Some escaping prisoners had also been

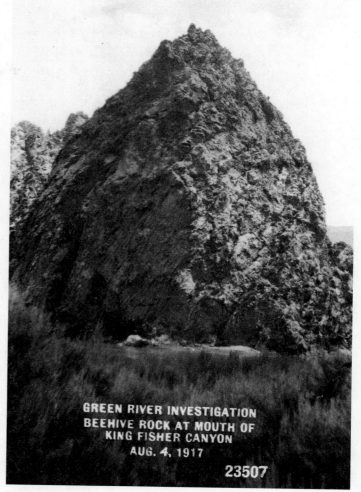

Beehive Rock, 1917.

traced to the mountains in this direction; then all tracks had ceased. [A rancher] asked us to help him swim some of his horses across the river. He said the high water had taken out his own boat. The horses were rounded up in a mountain-hidden valley and driven into the water ahead of the boat. After securing the horses, [his] welcome seemed to turn to suspicion and he questioned our reasons for being there, wanting to know what we could find in that wild country to interest us. [Later they were told that] [o]ur former host . . . had committed many depredations and had served one term for cattle stealing.[25]

This area was also the site of a campground, developed by the Civilian Conservation Corps during the Great Depression.[26] In 1947, when Norm Nevills stopped there for a day, he saw benches, tables, campfire rings, water hydrants, and another bridge across the river.

At this point the river had cut to the core of the Uintas. It swung to the east and continued along the very spine of the mountains. Dellenbaugh summed up the whole series: "Flaming Gorge is the gateway, Horseshoe the vestibule, and Kingfisher the antechamber to the whole grand series."[27] Below Hideout Flat, however, travelers had little time to admire the beauty of the canyons, for this was where the real rapids began.

Red Canyon

The core of the Uinta Mountains is made of the some of the oldest rocks on earth, the Uinta Mountain Quartzite. This ancient rock, some billions of years old, contains a great deal of iron and thus is deep red, lending the towering walls of Red Canyon a gloomy air. River runners know a simple equation: hard rock equals hard rapids. The side canyons were steep and narrow, and boulders washed out into the river

tended to stay put. Red Canyon also has the greatest total fall of any of the Green River canyons: 360 feet in 31 miles or 11.6 feet per mile.[28] As a result, the rapids started almost as soon as travelers entered Red Canyon and did not let up until the head of Browns Park. Everyone dismissed Powell's hyperbole about the rapids in Horseshoe and Kingfisher Canyons, but Red Canyon had plenty of real rapids. In 1896 Nathaniel Galloway—who had already run all of the Green and had been through Cataract Canyon on the Colorado by this time—and William Richmond met in Red Canyon and decided to run the whole river together, through the Grand Canyon. In a newspaper article written when they were about halfway through, Red Canyon, "which they say is the worst to get through between [Moab, Utah] and their starting point," was the one place they both remembered.[29]

There were four rapids in the first three miles; for experienced river runners like Don Hatch, Bert Loper, and Norm Nevills, they were just fun and splashy; for those who had never run rapids before, they were terrifying. Especially in the days of wooden boats, which could be smashed against a boulder, leaving the crew stranded or worse, the roaring water in Red Canyon was intimidating. If the water was high in the spring, the current was fast, demanding quick decisions. In the fall, when many early river runners preferred to go, the rapids became narrow, rocky chicanes. River runners quickly adopted inflatable rubber rafts when they became available in the years immediately after World War II. These craft made running rocky rapids such as those in Red Canyon much less threatening—if the raft hit a rock, it just bounced off. But they did not become commonly available until the late 1940s. Even in a rubber raft river runners approached Red Canyon with caution, for it had a fearsome reputation among boaters. Rafts had their own hazards (they could wrap themselves around a rock), but they were in use for only a few years before Red Canyon's rapids were silenced forever by the waters of Flaming Gorge Reservoir.

Fearing damage to his boats on his two voyages in the rocky Red Canyon rapids, John Wesley Powell lined almost every rapid in the whole canyon (unloading the boats and letting them down alongside the river with ropes while carrying equipment and supplies on foot along the side), to the disgust of his grumbling crews. In 1869 Powell's crews had suffered a devastating mishap when the *No Name* was wrecked in what he dubbed Disaster Falls in the Canyon of Lodore, downstream from Red Canyon. With that disaster in the back of his mind, Powell was anxious when his expedition once again approached Red Canyon in 1871. And he was right to be concerned: even though his 1869 crews passed through the upper end of Red Canyon without accident, in 1871 things turned out very differently. Without a little bit of luck, the ending could have been tragic.

On June 2, 1871, shortly after the party broke camp at the end of Kingfisher Canyon and headed downriver, the strong currents and swift water proved to be too much. Frederick Dellenbaugh was in the *Emma Dean* with Jack Hillers and Major Powell when the boat shot into an S-curve and was dashed against the righthand wall. One of the oarlocks manned by Hillers was torn off, leaving them only one set of oars in the hands of Dellenbaugh, the youngest member of the party at seventeen. He was able to get the boat to shore safely. Upstream was the *Nellie Powell*, with Almon Harris Thompson (the second-in-command), John F. Steward, Francis Bishop, and Frank Richardson on board. Dellenbaugh, Hillers, and Powell watched with horror as the *Nellie Powell* struck the wall and capsized. Bishop told the tale in his journal:

Today we start out for a run of a series of rapids and we know not what shall be. I expect we will get a ducking. Noon. Well! We have got it—the ducking I mean, and the way we got it was thusly. In the second rapid, we shipped pretty near a barrel of water, and stopped to bail out. All being ready, we pulled out and in about 15 minutes we came to a sharp bend and in the bend a strong current which set over to the west side. Our boat was caught and made it impossible for us to head down stream, and hurled us bang against the rocks, knocking a hole in her side and rolling the "*Nellie Powell*" upside down and necessitating an abrupt disembarking of the crew of the said "*Nellie P.*" For a few minutes things were pretty lively. We lost our camp kettle, sponge, and my compass, but no one got wet. I sprang to the rope and then on to the rocks giving it a twist around a rock to hold her from going down the stream. With a sharp strong pull up the bank she gradually righted up and floated four or five inches above water with her middle hatches full. We hauled her in and bailed out and commenced to repair . . . In about an hour and a half we got started again and ran down to the other boats.[30]

Bishop made light of a very serious situation; Richardson had been thrown out and trapped under the boat and had to be rescued by Thompson. The other boats could not come back to help them because the walls came right down to the river. One side of the boat was smashed; but "all being born mechanics," they were able to rebuild it on the spot.[31] In the meantime the final boat, *Canonita*, had made it through safely but had shipped a great deal of water. Powell, worried about a repeat of the wreck at Disaster Falls two years before, climbed the cliffs and hurried back upstream to see if he could tell what was happening; when he saw the boat ashore and being repaired, he no doubt breathed a huge sigh of relief. The two creeks right below the place where the accident occurred were named Kettle and Compass Creeks, to commemorate those lost articles, but were later renamed Trail and Allen Creeks. The party continued on its way, shaken and much more cautious.

In the ensuing years knowledge of the dangers in Red Canyon, as well as skill at running rapids, became more widespread. Later river travelers were more prepared for the fast water in Red Canyon. Even for an experienced boatman in an inflatable raft like Harry Aleson, though, it could be an exhilarating ride. Marjorie Steurt, a passenger on one of Aleson's river trips, left a breathless account:

Red Canyon seems to be the start of the rapids. Harry stands up and tries to make a quick calculation of where to go through. Once he makes his choice there is no turning back. First comes a deceptively smooth lake. Then the water, still smooth, starts to flow faster and faster. Finally it erupts in foam on a rock and we go shooting down a narrow channel barely wide enough for the boat. A rock looms high out of the water directly ahead of us and Harry, with a deft flip of the oar sends us around it, only to scrape on a rock we had not seen. Safely over that we go shooting down a zig-zag course where every minutes we think we are going to pile up on the rocks. Finally we are through. I let out a whoop. Harry relaxes. Charles just sits and smiles.[32]

Carter Creek
But Red Canyon was not all gloomy red walls, growling rapids, and looming disaster; in many places clear mountain streams came cascading into the main channel. These locations were usually open, sun-filled, and shaded by

tall fir and pine trees. The streams were full of tasty trout. The area had few sandy beaches like those on the lower Green or the Colorado, but soft grass made up for the lack. One of the favorite camps was at the mouth of Carter Creek, named for Judge William Carter of Fort Bridger. An article in the *Sierra Club Bulletin* in 1960 made it sound very inviting: "After a short run of about six miles we arrive at Carter Creek tributary, a beautiful trout stream. Here in the pine country surrounded by high mountains and red cliffs we will make our first camp. A layover day will give the fishermen an opportunity to try their skill."[33] Ralf Woolley was entranced with Carter Creek:

> Carter Creek flows in a rugged gorge with steep walls, entering the Green River from the south. The stream carried about 100 or 125 second-feet of clear, cold water at the time of our visit and seemed to be very well stocked with mountain trout. Thirty-five fine trout were caught during the two or three hours before dark . . . The camp at Carter Creek was a beautiful spot in a cluster of pine trees, with a fine cold spring of sparkling water close at hand for drinking water.[34]

Cid Ricketts Sumner, who camped at Carter Creek in 1955, was inspired almost to poetry:

> The sun, not yet quite cut off by the towering cliff opposite, was still shining down here. By a cleft in this wall and a wooded

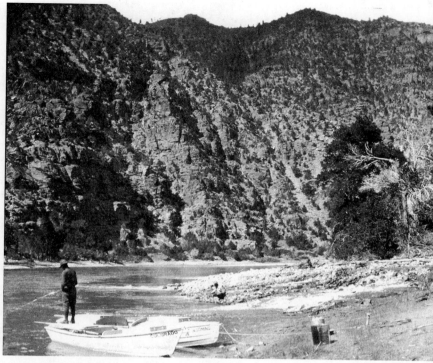

Mouth of Carter Creek.

widening, a clear rushing stream dashed down over a tumble of rocks to join the river. Tall pines glinted silver and green, their straight trunks rosied by the sun. The ground sloped gently back to a more level spot under the trees where a rough table had been set, a board bench alongside it, for others had camped here. Carter Creek. I shall never think of it but with a sense of completion, of fulfillment, as if here at last I had arrived at perfection.[35]

Another pleasant aspect of Red Canyon was the plentiful wildlife. Many travelers report seeing deer, elk, beaver, and river otters. Deer

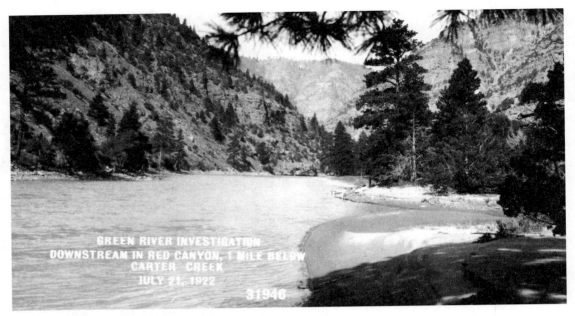

Mouth of Eagle Creek, Red Canyon.

were especially plentiful; in 1940 Bert Loper noted: "I expect that we saw 125 deer in red canyon [*sic*] and . . . about a million young geese and ducks."[36] Ken Sleight, who ran a few river trips for hunters as the dam was being built, remembered deer being so thick in the canyons that he had to make a rule that his clients had to wait to get off the boat before shooting a deer; otherwise, he said, it was like shooting fish in a barrel.[37]

But even after camping at a beautiful place like Carter Creek—and Red Canyon had many other such places—travelers still had rapids to run, and the sound of swift water was ever present. One of the classic accounts of adventure in Red Canyon involves two young men from St. Louis. Tom Martin, a graduate of Annapolis and veteran of the Spanish–American War, and his friend Jules W. Woodward were both members of the Missouri Athletic Club and expert swimmers. They planned to explore the remote canyons of the Green and Colorado Rivers together all the way to the Gulf of California. They felt ready, as described in an article in the *St. Louis Republic*:

> Martin and Woodward are taking no rash risks. Both are trained athletes and both are accustomed to risks on land and water. They are likely to spend a good deal of time in the water of the Colorado, righting their boat after it has been capsized. As swimmers they are prepared this by long training, part of which was swimming in water full of floating ice during

their excursion on the Niangua River in February, 1908. Just before starting from Green River for the 2,000-mile journey to the Gulf of California, Woodward wrote his brother that all preparation had been made for the greatest trip of his life . . . these preparations seem to leave nothing that is needed for anticipating and overcoming the worst dangers. Their boat, specially made by the St. Louis Boat and Engine company, is 18 feet long, clinker built, to draw six inches when fully loaded. As a most important feature, it has two mammoth air tanks of galvanized iron, placed one at each end, so that it will not sink when overturned. In the expectation that it will be frequently overturned, it has also two compartments of galvanized iron, watertight and airtight, for carrying matches, ammunition and other necessaries which might be ruined by contact with water. The provisions for the five months the adventurers expect to spend on the river before reaching the Gulf of California from Wyoming, are mostly in tins, tied to the boat, so that they will not be lost in any upset . . . It means now what the old story tellers meant when they wrote of getting beyond the bounds of the world and passing the narrow channels where death lies on one side and destruction on the other, with passage only for those who can keep the middle way between, without shrinking form danger on either side.[38]

The story concluded on an ominous note: "Those who descend the full as the Colorado pours its waters into the Grand Canyon, leave all hope behind, except the winning hope with which the St. Louis expedition enters the canyon; the hope of courage, trained to control through presence of mind until every nerve and fiber of the body obeys it." The article turned out to be prescient. They had covered about eighty miles and were somewhere in Red Canyon when their boat was "destroyed in the swift current [when] one of the oarlocks was broken and the craft became unmanageable in the turbulent water." As the boat capsized, both men were thrown into the water and barely made it to shore, with only the clothes on their backs. Their specially made boat and all of their carefully packed food and equipment was lost. After three days wandering in the canyons, they made their way out to an abandoned cabin where they found matches and flour. They met an Indian who gave them an old pair of pants to tear up to make coverings for their bare feet and finally walked a further thirty miles to Linwood.[39]

When the Kolb brothers started on a similar voyage two years later, the sad tale of the two young men from St. Louis was no doubt told to them with relish by the wags in Green River. Ellsworth reflected on it in his book: "After two weeks treatment in hospital in Green River City they were partially restored to health. Quite likely they spent many of the long hours of their convalescence on the river bank, or on the little island, watching the unruffled stream glide underneath the cottonwoods."[40]

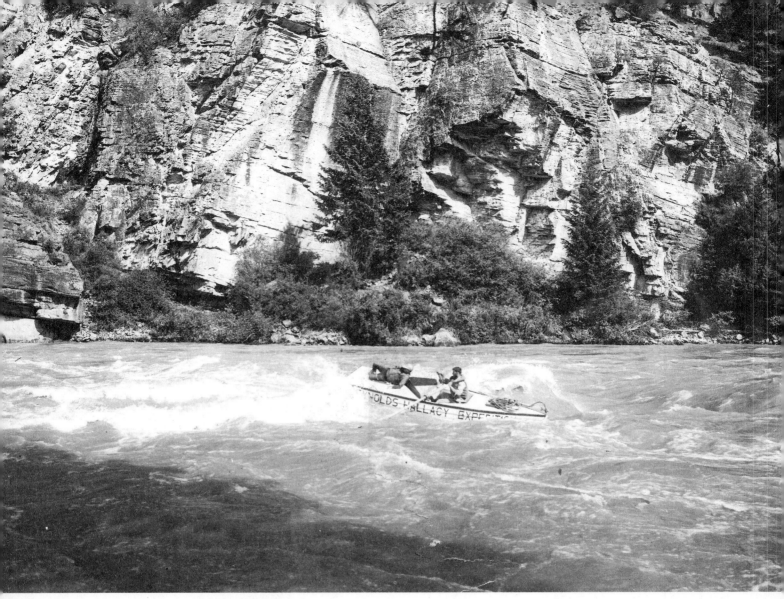

Skull Creek Rapid, 1950.

Skull Creek Rapid

It's impossible to tell where Martin and Wood-ward lost their boat, but it could have been Skull Creek, one of the few named rapids in Red Canyon. Big rocks in the channel meant big holes and waves in high water, and it was easy to capsize a boat there. Ralf Woolley described Skull Creek as "the roughest water thus far encountered . . . This rapid was more than a half mile long, comprising a close succession of swift currents. The stream channel is spotted with huge boulders. Many of them are submerged only a few inches and although not visible thru the muddy water they were marked by eddys."[41] Helen Kendall, on the river with Georgie White in 1960, described Skull Creek as a long rocky rapid with multiple channels: "Shut off motor and John rowed thru the rapids, swing thru a very narrow channel to keep the boats from hitting the cliff. A natural dam of round rocks separates the two channels and the one on the right looks much higher than the one on the left which we are in. Went thru another riffle while watching the two channels."[42]

Skull Creek was likely the place where one of the most famous incidents in Red Canyon occurred, the drowning of Theodore Hook of Green River City in 1869. Hook, a land speculator and prospector, knew of John Wesley Powell's planned voyage down the Green and decided to beat him to what Hook was sure were rich deposits of minerals. He and several companions, including Jesse Ewing, later to become a permanent resident of Browns Park, left secretly in the dead of night to see for themselves before any dude from back East beat them to it. Accounts vary as to their craft; most sources say that they were in two or three small skiffs, while another claims that it was a raft made of railroad ties. In any case, the vessels must not have been adequate for the task, for at one point the boat Hook was in "suddenly dropped out of sight, plunging into a foaming whirlpool." It came out upside down with Hook's companion holding on for dear life. The other boats made it to shore while Hook climbed up on a rock in the middle of the river. Before the others could rescue him,

he jumped back into the river to swim to the side and promptly disappeared. His body was found some distance downstream and was buried in Browns Park.[43]

Frederick Dellenbaugh passed the site of the accident two years later and noted: "Their abandoned boats, flat-bottomed and inadequate, still lay half-buried in sand on the left-hand bank, and not far off on a sandy knoll was the grave of the unfortunate leader marked by a pine board set up, with his name painted on it. Old sacks, ropes, oars, etc., emphasized the completeness of the disaster."[44]

Like so many legends of the Old West, this one comes in many different versions. Several place this as happening in 1868, but there is little doubt that the accident occurred in 1869, based on contemporary newspaper stories that reported the death of Hook, who was a well-known citizen of early Wyoming. Some of those same newspaper stories say that the party had as many as fifteen members in no fewer than five boats. Dellenbaugh, Thompson, Jones, and Clem Powell, of Powell's 1871 crew, refer to two boats. Dellenbaugh says that Hook drowned above Ashley Falls and was buried on the spot, even noting the grave and board that marked it (as quoted above). None of the other crew members refer to a grave, however, and a great deal of local tradition as well as statements made at the time by other members of Powell's second crew (such as Steven Vandiver Jones and Walter Clement Powell) place Hook's grave in Browns Park.

At this point it seems safe to say that all of

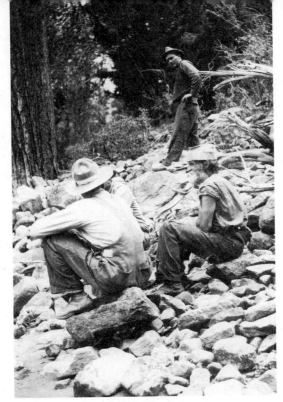

Amos Hill, the "Hermit of Red Canyon," 1922.

mouth of the short, steep Jarvies Canyon, named for that ill-fated resident of Browns Park. The river made a hairpin turn around Gold Point and passed the mouths of Trail Creek and Allen Creek.[47] In 1922 Ralf Woolley was surprised to find a hermit living there in a hole in the ground. His name was Amos Hill:

The hermit was at home, and he was as much surprised to see the visitors as they were to see him. He gave his name as Amos Hill and said that he was 71 years old and had lived in the canyon about 20 years. His house or hovel was a crude tepee of boards over a small hole in the ground. It was hardly big enough for one person but might be classed as a good-sized dog kennel. His wardrobe was as meager as the house, consisting of a piece of dirty canvas with a hole cut in the middle for his head to pass through, a ragged pair of overalls, and a unique pair of shoes with soles of large pieces of cowhide about 15 inches long with the hair on the bottom side and uppers apparently cut from old rubber boots and laced to the soles with rawhide strings. It was about noon when the party reached this place, and Mr. Hill was invited to lunch. He conversed freely. Among other things he claimed to have gone through the Green River canyons on a raft, taking a horse with him—a feat which one who has been through the canyons would be justified in believing impossible.[48]

these accounts contain some truth: Hook did indeed drown above Ashley Falls, perhaps in Skull Creek Rapid, and his body was found some distance downstream and buried near what would later become the Jarvie Ranch in Browns Park.[45] According to George Young Bradley, who was with Powell in 1869, yet another small party of two prospectors in a single boat started before Powell; they floated to below Ashley Falls, left the river, and walked out. Nor was Hook the only victim of Skull Creek; in 1917, Bert Loper was told, a man by the name of Green drowned there trying to cross the river.[46]

The Hermit of Red Canyon
Just below Skull Creek, the river passed the

Hill, who had been there since about 1900, had dug ditches to divert Trail and Allen Creeks so that he could grow a little alfalfa, corn, and vegetables. He was apparently a "cantankerous man" who had gotten into several fights that resulted in charges and was now hiding out from the law. Woolley was one of the last people to see his canyon hovel, for Hill was not there in 1926 when the Todd–Page party passed by; perhaps the canyons had gotten too crowded for him.[49]

The mouth of Trail Creek was also one of William Purdy's favorite camps, not least because of a huge chokecherry bush that he would always visit in season. Purdy noted that he could fill two large buckets with chokecherries every year. Naturally, it also had other visitors. Once Purdy, the principal at the school in Manila, who had run Red Canyon "dozens of times," camped there with a party of friends. It was a warm night with a beautiful full moon; Purdy was not sleepy as the evening wound down, so he went for a walk. Just outside the circle of light cast by their big fire, he came face to face with a "huge black bear." Shaken, Purdy went back to camp and warned the others, who were sleeping by the fire. One friend, however, who had a habit of sleeping in the nude, had made his bed right by the bushes on a small terrace. He scoffed at Purdy: "No bear is going to make me get out of bed." Just then the bushes rattled and out came not one

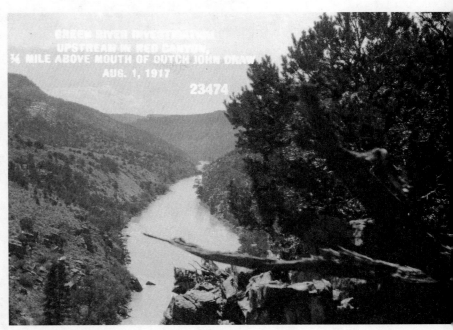

Near Dutch John Draw.

but five bears. "It was like Yellowstone," Purdy later recalled. The friend closest to the bears jumped out of his sleeping bag and ran naked toward the river, "his bare ass shining in the moonlight," leaving the others convulsed with laughter.[50]

From the mouth of Trail Creek a few miles of swift water ran between high canyon walls. By this point every river traveler on the Green was looking ahead with anticipation and even dread for the one rapid everyone had heard of: Ashley Falls. So in the next chapter we'll pause in our journey on the Green River to consider this famous rapid.

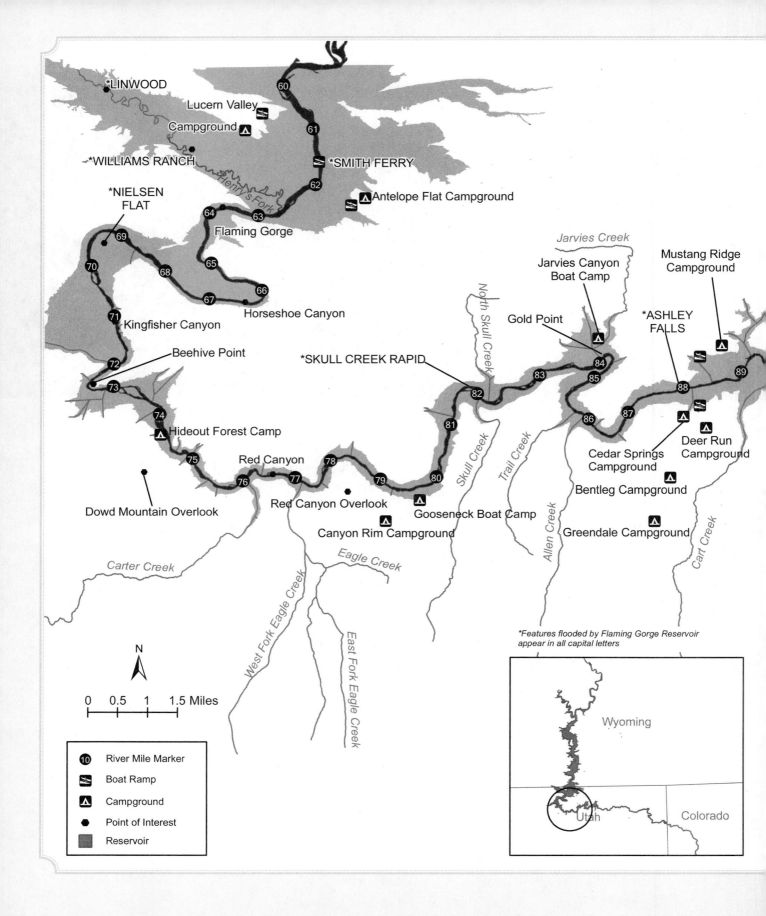

*LINWOOD

Lucern Valley
Campground ⛺

*WILLIAMS RANCH

*NIELSEN
FLAT

*SMITH FERRY

⛺ Antelope Flat Campground

Flaming Gorge

Horseshoe Canyon

Kingfisher Canyon

Beehive Point

*SKULL CREEK RAPID

Jarvies Canyon
Boat Camp

Gold Point

Jarvies Creek

Mustang Ridge
Campground

*ASHLEY
FALLS

North Skull Creek

⛺ Hideout Forest Camp

Red Canyon

Dowd Mountain Overlook

Red Canyon Overlook

⛺ Canyon Rim Campground

Gooseneck Boat Camp

Skull Creek

Trail Creek

Cedar Springs
Campground

Bentleg Campground

Greendale Campground

Deer Run
Campground

Allen Creek

Cart Creek

Carter Creek

Eagle Creek

West Fork Eagle Creek

East Fork Eagle Creek

*Features flooded by Flaming Gorge Reservoir
appear in all capital letters

N

0   0.5   1   1.5 Miles

🔟 River Mile Marker

≋ Boat Ramp

⛺ Campground

⬢ Point of Interest

▨ Reservoir

Wyoming

Utah

Colorado

ASHLEY FALLS

We ran along on still water, with a vague feeling of trouble ahead, for about two miles, when, turning an abrupt corner, we came in sight of the first fall about three hundred yards below us ... [The crew] found a fall of about ten feet in twenty-five. There is a nearly square rock in the middle of the stream about twenty-five by thirty feet, the top fifteen feet above the water. There are many smaller ones all the way across, placed in such a manner that the fall is broken into steps, two on the east side, three on the west. We all saw that a portage would have to be made here.

—JOHN COLTON (JACK) SUMNER, 1869

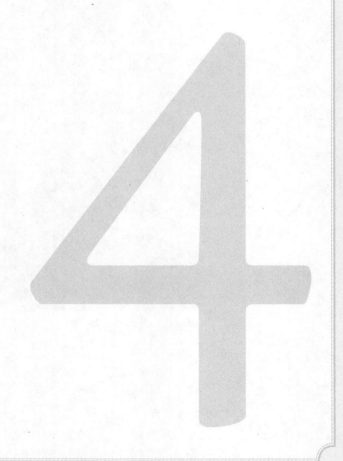

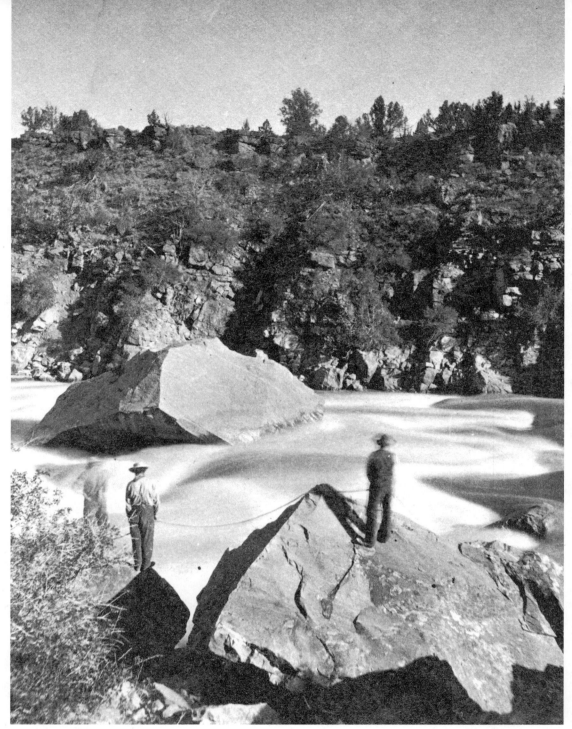

Powell lining Ashley Falls, 1871.

Ashley Falls deserves its own chapter, for no other rapid looms as large in the history of the Green River. Even Red Creek, the big rapids in the Canyon of Lodore like Disaster Falls and Hells Half Mile, and all other rapids along the Green, many of which are much more difficult to navigate, did not have the same impact as Ashley Falls did. Legends grew up around the falls; it was often said that Ashley had met with disaster there in varying ways. In many stories this somehow became conflated with the legend of the dreaded Green River Suck. In the early days of travel on the Green, no other rapid was written about so often or anticipated with such anxiety and dread as Ashley Falls. In 1824 William Ashley was the first known person to pass it. William Manly and no doubt some others were there in 1849. Manly left the first written record of what would become known as Ashley Falls:

> Just before night we came to a place where some huge rocks as large as cabins had fallen down from the mountain, completely filling up the river bed, and making it completely impassible for our boat. We unloaded it and while the boys held the stern line, I took off my clothes and pushed the boat out into the torrent which ran around the rock, letting them pay the line out slowly till it was just right. Then I said out to "Let Go!" and away it dashed. I grasped the bow line, and at the first chance jumped overboard and got to shore.[1]

Manly was the first, but not the last, to wonder at the name he saw painted on the rocks above the rapid:

> While I was looking up toward the mountain top, and along down the rocky wall, I saw a smooth place about fifty feet above where the great rocks had broken out, and there, painted in large black letters, were the words "ASHLEY, 1824 [sic]." This was the first real evidence we had of the presence of a white man in this wild place.[2]

Neither Ashley nor Manly recorded any great difficulty in getting past Ashley Falls; they just carried their boats around it. But their accounts were not published until years later.[3] In the ensuing years a series of legends somehow grew up around Ashley Falls, making it seem like a modern Scylla and Charybdis with a portal inscribed "Abandon all hope, ye who enter here." Dellenbaugh, writing about Ashley and relying on the unreliable Jim Beckwourth, spins a horrifying tale of disaster, death, and even cannibalism:

> They took along few provisions, expecting to find beaver plentiful to the end of the canyon, but after a few miles the beaver were absent, and, having preserved none of the meat, the party began to suffer for food. They were six days without eating, and, the high precipitous walls, running ever on and on, they became disheartened, or, in the Western phrase, "demoralized," and proposed to cast lots to find which should make food for the others, a proposition which horrified Ashley, and he begged them to hold out longer, assuring them that the walls must soon break and enable them to escape.[4]

Powell himself was certainly concerned about this and took as an omen the stories current in the town of Green River about the Green River Suck and trappers' tales of Ashley's supposed hardships. "The word 'Ashley' is a warning to us, and we resolve on great caution. Ashley Falls is the name we give to the cataract."[5]

No wonder so many early river travelers fretted about Ashley Falls long before they reached it. Even as late at the 1930s Ashley Falls was viewed with trepidation. Russell Frazier, a passenger with Bus Hatch on a 1937 trip, wrote: "We were shortly to enter Red Canyon, and the treacherous Ashley Falls. Here it was, we learned with misgiving, that

in 1825 [*sic*: 1824], out of Col. Ashley's party of nine, seven were drowned. The prospects looked ominous. The river was becoming narrower and faster as it flowed through canyons 1500 to 2000 feet deep. Then the roar of distant rapids announced with no uncertainty that we were in for Ashley Falls."[6] The Kolb brothers in 1911 considered Ashley Falls such a significant milestone that they waited until they were safely below it to name their boats.[7]

Ashley Falls certainly looked impressive. The towering thousand-foot canyon walls had given way to much lower ones, with rolling hills above. At some point in the past huge boulders had fallen off the walls and choked the channel, forming Ashley Falls. The total drop in the rapid is unrecorded, but from photographs it appears to be about ten vertical feet in a very short distance. Almon Harris Thompson, with Powell in 1871, thought that this was very recent: "[T]he cliff on the left has fallen within perhaps 50 years and filled in the left bank, narrowing the river 1/3 and thrown high blocks across the stream, damming it so that the river is quiet for a half a mile above."[8] No matter when it occurred, this actually made Ashley Falls unique. Virtually every other rapid in Red Canyon—or in any canyon—is formed when boulders are washed down a side canyon into the mail channel; there was no side canyon at Ashley Falls. The rock in the middle was literally the size of a house; the ones on either side the size of wagons. The rocks blocking the channel made getting past Ashley Falls difficult, whether by lining (holding onto the unloaded boats by ropes and carrying equipment and supplies on foot) or portaging or in a boat. Lining was all but impossible on the right side because of the cliff and grueling on the left side because of the size of the boulders. George Bradley, with Powell on his pioneering 1869 voyage, lamented the amount of work facing them: "[B]ut we have to carry the rations around on our back, and as the shore is filled with huge bowlders [sic] recently fallen from the mountain, we shall have a hard day's work, to get all around tomorrow for each of the three large boats has over 2000 lbs. baggage."[9] Both Bradley and Jack Sumner commented on the Ashley inscription, and Sumner at least got the date 1825 right.

It had not gotten any easier when Powell returned for his 1871 expedition two years later, for his boats and supplies were essentially the same. Stephen Vandiver Jones, the assistant topographer for the party, left the best description of the falls:

> For half a mile above the fall the river is quiet as if preparing for the leap. At the head it is divided into 2 streams by a rock of 50 or 60 tons weight that has fallen into the stream. The water on the right falls almost vertically about 4 or 5 feet breaking into foam, throwing the spray to the height of several feet. The stream on the left falls about the same distance but is less broken over both precipices. The river is full of sunken rocks, and nearly precipitous cliffs rise on each side to near 400 feet,

composed of Red Sandstone [sic]. The roar of the falls can be heard nearly a mile above. The course of the river is nearly east, and the rays of the setting sun formed a beautiful rainbow at the lower end of the rocks in the middle of the stream.[10]

Just like the previous expeditions, Powell's men did not feel they could run Ashley Falls, so they laboriously portaged all their supplies and one boat, the *Emma Dean* (which weighed close to a ton), over the rocks. Deciding that this was too much work they tried to line the next boat but quickly ran into trouble trying to let the *Canonita* down with ropes, as Jones describes: "When she struck the fall and the stern line was cast loose, she shot through like lightning, careened, filled, jerked the line through my hands, entangled in Fred's [Dellenbaugh's] feet, and came near drawing him into the water."[11]

John F. Steward, another crew member, described what happened after the boat shot over the fall: "Although with bow upstream, the pressure was so great that she broke away. By mere luck some of the boys seized the stern rope and made it sufficiently fast to hold her. She pounded against the rocks until I jumped to the boat from the rocks above, and secured the rope to her bow again, but with much difficulty, yet without being thrown out."[12]

Walter Clement Powell, a young nephew of John Wesley Powell, said that the *Canonita* turned over twice, but none of the other accounts mention this.

At any rate, it was obvious that lining past Ashley Falls was more risk than the party was willing to accept, so the final boat, the *Nellie Powell*, was lifted out of the water and hauled by hand over the boulder field, as Frederick Dellenbaugh, the youngest member of the party, described: "[W]e resorted to sliding and carrying the *Nell* over the rocks as we had done with the *Dean*, certain that sleep and food would wipe out our weariness, but not injury to the boats which must be avoided by all means in our power. By the time we had placed the *Nell* beside the other boats at the bottom it was sunset and too late to do anything but make a camp."[13]

Interestingly, and perhaps because of the excitement and labor of lining and portaging, none of these journal-keepers on this voyage save one commented on the Ashley inscription on the left wall. Dellenbaugh did take time out to find Ashley's inscription, going out of his way during one portage trip to view the name and make a detailed drawing. The observant Dellenbaugh also recorded a detailed description: "On one of my trips over the rocks with cargo I made a slight detour on the return to see the boulder where the Major had discovered Ashley's name with a date. The letters were in black, just under a slight projection and were surprisingly distinct considering the forty-six years of exposure. The '2' was illegible and looked like a '3.' None of our party seemed to know that it could have been only a '2' for by the year 1835 Ashley had sold out and had given up the fur business in the mountains."[14]

More important than any descriptions of the rapid, though, were the views of Ashley Falls taken by E. O. Beaman, the expedition photographer, as the others lined and portaged the boats. These were the first photographs ever taken of the rapid. With the glass-plate cameras of the day, Beaman was forced to take long exposures; the high water of June, flowing through the rocks, appears like a smooth wave, giving Ashley Falls an ethereal, haunted look.

For the rest of the nineteenth century Ashley Falls was left mostly to itself, the water rising and falling in response to the seasons as it had for uncounted millennia. The Uinta Mountains and Red Canyon were frequented only by Native Americans and outlaws, since the roads over the mountains tended to bypass Red Canyon. Sometime in the late 1800s, Nathaniel Galloway, a trapper and orchard-keeper from Vernal, Utah, started navigating the upper Green in boats of his own design: light, flat-bottomed skiffs that were very maneuverable and designed to run rapids. Galloway was a taciturn man and rarely commented in his brief journals on the canyons he traveled through and the rapids he passed, but he was probably the first person who actually ran, rather than portaged or lined, Ashley Falls.[15] The first run of Ashley Falls was not recorded until 1896, when George Flavell ran the entire river in his little punt *Panthon* with a companion, Ramon Montéz. He noted: "One place the river was completely dammed up with boulders which caused a falls of four feet, the widest passage being ten feet. That was enough for

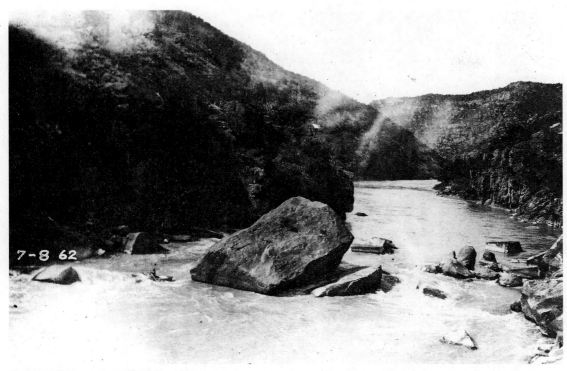

Nathaniel Galloway in Ashley Falls, 1909.

the *PANTHON*, so we passed on."[16] Galloway himself wrote about the rapid in the journal he kept during the Galloway–Stone expedition of 1909. Reaching Ashley Falls in September's low water, Galloway and Julius Stone scouted it and then ran it with no real problems. This description comes from the journal he kept on the 1909 trip:

> After examination I decide to run all the boats thru the center channel running directly towards the large cubelar [*sic*] rock in the center. This channel is so narrow at the entrance that one must fold the oars back by the side of the boat as soon as the first rocks are passed. One has but about 15 ft. to direct the boat to prevent dashing into the large rock. I decide to run all the boats because the other men have had but little experience in rapids. But after running two of the boats Mr. Stone decides to run his own boat, following me with the 3rd boat. But on starting in to the rapid Mr. Stone lost one of his oar locks and came thru with but one oar without a mishap.[17]

Two years passed before more river travelers braved Ashley Falls. Emery and Ellsworth Kolb had a photo studio on the rim of

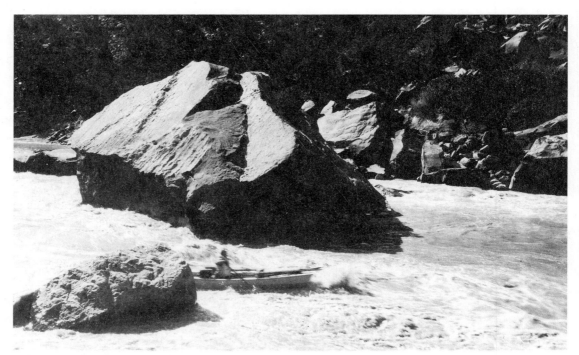

Bert Loper running Ashley Falls, 1922.

the Grand Canyon and were veterans of many adventures; but this was the first time they had attempted a long river voyage. They reached Ashley Falls in late September, when the water was low. This was their first taste of the hundreds of rapids to come. Seeing the tumult of rocks and water made them remember those warnings from the people in Green River:

At 2:30 PM we reached Ashley Falls, a rapid we had been expecting to see for some time . . . A dozen immense rocks had fallen from the cliff on the left, almost completely blocking the channel—or so it seemed from one point of view. But there was a crooked channel, not more than twelve feet wide in places, through which the water shot like a stream from a nozzle. We wanted a motion picture of our dash through the chute. But the location for the camera was hard to secure, for a sheer bank of rock or low wall prevented us from climbing out on the right side. We overcame this by landing on a little bank at the base of the wall and by dropping a boat down with a line to the head of the rapid, where a break occurred in the wall . . . Almost before I knew it I was in the narrow channel, so close to the right rock that I had to ship that oar, and pull all together on the left one. As soon as I was through I made a few quick strokes, but the current was too strong for me; and a corner of the stern struck with a bang when I was almost clear. She paused as a wave rolled over the decks, then rose quickly; a side current caught the boat, whirling it around, and the bow struck. I was still pulling with all my might, but everything happened so quickly with the boat whirling first this way, then that— that my efforts were almost useless. But after that second strike I did get in a few strokes, and pulled into the quiet pool below the line of boulders. Emery held his boat in better position than I had done, and it looked for a while as if he would make it. But the EDITH struck on the stern, much as mine had done. Then he pulled clear and joined me in the shelter of the large rock, as cool and smiling as if he had been rowing on a mill-pond.[18]

The next written account of Ashley Falls comes from the 1922 USGS dam site survey. They reached Ashley Falls on July 24, after stopping just upriver at Trail Creek to visit with the "Hermit of Red Canyon," Amos Hill. The hermit warned them about Ashley Falls; but Loper, who had never run the rapid but was one of the most experienced boatmen of his day, was not deterred. After scouting the rapid, Loper, H. Elwyn Blake, and Leigh Lint "ran their own boats through," and "[b]y 4:30 Ashley Falls was behind us." Even though he left only a very brief description of the rapid, Woolley, who was also the trip's photographer,

took several fine views of Ashley Falls with his panorama camera.[19]

Loper himself never came back to Ashley Falls, but Blake did just a few years later.[20] In 1926 a party of young college men from Princeton—F. Lemoyne Page, Web Todd, and Ogden "Og" West—came out to the rugged Green River for a vacation. They hired Blake as their guide; with a friend of Blake's, Curley Hale, as camp help, they started just above Flaming Gorge on July 23, 1926. They reached Ashley Falls the next morning. For Blake, who by this point had been a boatman on the San Juan River, Green River, Cataract Canyon, and Grand Canyon surveys, the rapid held little fear. After a "brief inspection" they ran both boats through fully loaded and with all passengers aboard. In any event, no mishaps occurred with the boats. "[T]hen something heretofore not dared was suggested: that we swim it!" All put on their life jackets, climbed back up through the rocks to the head of the rapid, and gaily floated through.[21]

The 1930s saw a great deal of change on the river, not the least of which was the increase in the number of river runners. Among these were the fun-loving Hatch brothers and associated friends and relatives, who started taking trips down the Green from Hideout Flats as early as 1931 but unfortunately left little account of their portage of Ashley Falls that year or of the trip they made with Dr. Russell Frazier in 1932. In the fall of 1937 solo boatman Buzz Holmstrom came to Ashley Falls, having heard a great deal about it from the good citizens of Green River, Wyoming. He reached it on the afternoon of October 8, 1937, and found that it was not nearly as bad as he had been led to believe. His greatest hazard was the low stage of the water:

Ashley F[alls] at 4:30—took two time ex[posures]—probably no good tho—ran without any trouble—altho close quarters—half mile below is a ford—just after I got the pict of falls I saw a pack-train crossing—I rowed down fast & talked to the men—4 of them & half dozen pack horses—they had driven a herd of cows from Vernal to Green R and this is the shortest route.[22]

Holmstrom was back the next year, along with a number of other parties; in fact, 1938 became the banner year for river-running parties down the Green, with no fewer than four separate groups on the river around the same time. With filmmaker Amos Burg, who was rowing his own inflatable raft, they reached Ashley Falls on September 7. There was quite a bit more water than the year before, but it made little difference to Buzz; by now he had over a thousand river miles under his boat and was on his way to becoming one of the best boatmen of his time.

4:50 Have arrived Ashley Falls & looked over—Amos is going to take MP [motion pictures] from Hi on L bank of me going & then I'll take his—more fall here than

before—but can go down right channel—instead of in middle as before—quite rough looking tho especially rock at foot on R—know more about that soon—will wear life pres[erver] anyway—saw Stone Coggs [Cogswell] & Galloway names on L—sky very dark—no good for color—not much color here anyway 5:30 All fine at the Falls—good side current pulls boat toward center big rock from R & sends it thru just rite—I didn't even get deck wet & Amos went thru just fine—Very strong current tho & if boat got out of position it would be very bad.[23]

Just a few days after Burg and Holmstrom passed Ashley Falls, another group arrived at the rapid: the de Colmont/de Seynes party, usually just known as the French kayakers. This trio consisted of Bernard de Colmont; his young wife, Geneviève; and their friend Antoine de Seynes. They had come all the way from France to run the Green River and Colorado in folding kayaks, and Ashley Falls was their first major rapid. Bernard, the most experienced boater of the group, ran all three kayaks through the rapid while Antoine and Geneviève filmed from the left shore.

At 11 o'clock, we arrive at Ashley Falls, the first serious rapids as described in the stories of other expeditions which preceded us. An enormous boulder surrounded by smaller boulders blocks the river. We land and go along the rocks on

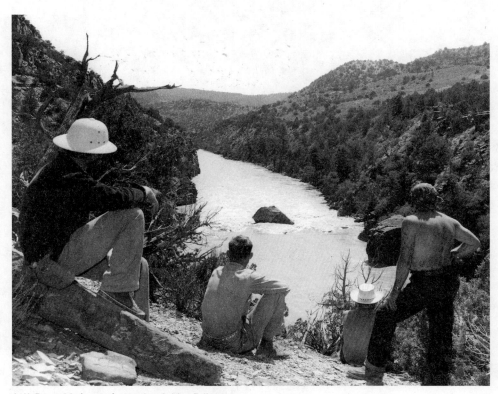

A. K. Reynolds (center) scouting Ashley Falls, 1950.

the bank to study the rapids. Bernard then decides to pass the three boats in succession, while Geneviève and I take photos and film . . . The only delicate point in these rapids is that the right route, which passes between two rocks, comes out right on the largest boulder that must be avoided and passed on the right.[24]

After Bernard had all three boats safely below the rapid, they camped just below. Geneviève later added their names to the growing "river register" that had been begun by William Ashley over a hundred years before.

Yet another party passed through Ashley Falls that year. The Lee Kay wildlife survey started from Hideout Flat a few days after the French kayakers passed by. Dr. Kay, however, was more interested in the fate of the vanished mountain sheep than in the rapids, historic or otherwise, and left no account of their run. Finally, Stewart Gardiner, a young man from Salt Lake City who was floating the river solo in a folding kayak just on a lark, ran Ashley Falls later that same year. Gardiner was a complete novice who had ordered his boat from a catalog. He decided to run the Green as a summer vacation and had his father drive him from

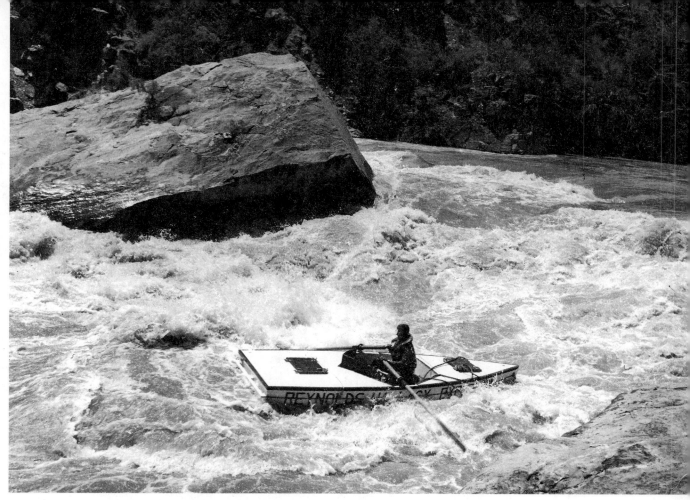

A. K. Reynolds running Ashley Falls, 1950.

Salt Lake City and drop him off. Starting from Hideout Flat, Gardiner came upon Ashley Falls soon after he started his trip and before he got the feel of his boat:

> Ashley Falls . . . had these huge, huge boulders that had fallen down into the river. It wasn't actually a fall. Ashley Falls is now covered by the reservoir. But originally there were these huge, huge boulders. I guess they must have been fifteen or twenty feet across. As you come into

where the water went by these rocks it was picking up speed. There wasn't a lot of big waves, but it was swift going through. You had to go through between some smaller rocks and heading right for this one big huge one. You just had to turn real sharp to get around it. I remember I just . . . missed that rock.[25]

During the 1940s Ashley Falls saw fewer river runners than in the previous decades, but it was not because of lack of interest in the

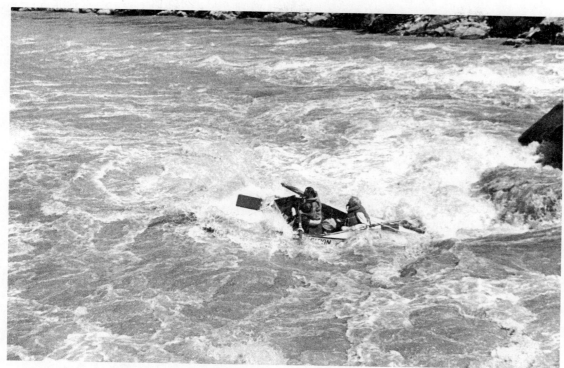

Norm Nevills running Ashley Falls, 1947.

river. Rationing during World War II made gas, tires, and oil hard to come by; river runners, like everyone else, were often unable to go where they wanted because of the restrictions on travel. Before the war, pioneer commercial river outfitter Norman Nevills of Mexican Hat, Utah, took an expedition down the Green and Colorado Rivers, all the way from Green River, Utah, through the Grand Canyon. Nevills ran the upper Green, and hence Ashley Falls, first in 1940 and again in 1947 and 1949. In this description of the first run, he obviously put more time into rigging a sling to paint his name on the river register than he did in worrying about the rapid:

MILE 292. ASHLEY FALLS. After some study I decided to run thru on the left, with passengers. Its [*sic*] a bit tricky, tho not dangerous. With the landing of the *WEN*, look across river and see names of various parties on wall. Decide to cross over and put our names up too. Signal the *MEXICAN HAT* thru, then the *JOAN*. Doris and Larabee rode with me thru this rapid. Was quite a job to get the names up on a huge rock on the left bank. Had to work from a sling. Saw a good many names, including those of the Stone party. Our names, written under NEVILLS EXPEDITION 1940, are about 75' above the river, in white paint.[26]

In 1947, though, Nevills remembered that he had heard that Don Harris, a friend of his from Mexican Hat, Utah, had tried to run the left side and capsized; Harris didn't recover his boat until about thirty miles downstream. Perhaps wary because of that, Nevills lined two of his three boats then decided that was too much work, so "I run the *JOAN* right on through ASHLEY FALLS! Nothing to it."[27] Garth Marston, Dock's son and one of the boatmen on the trip, thought the same: unbeknownst to Nevills, he and one of the passengers hiked back upstream and then floated through the rapid in their life jackets, to the dismay of Nevills.

Virtually every river runner who traversed Red Canyon left an account of Ashley Falls, for it was the one place on the mind of all river runners. In his description, however, Norm Nevills brings up two interesting things about the rapid. First, it was the site of a long-standing river register, where many earlier travelers had painted or chiseled their names, starting with William Ashley in 1825, who left his name and the date on a boulder on the left above the rapid. Numerous later travelers followed his example: William Manly in 1849, the Galloway–Stone expedition in 1909, the Langley expedition with Bus Hatch in 1936, the French kayakers and Amos Burg and Buzz Holmstrom in 1938, Norm Nevills in 1940, and many more. A few photos of some of the inscriptions on the river register exist, and glimpses of them can be seen in films of runs through the rapid.

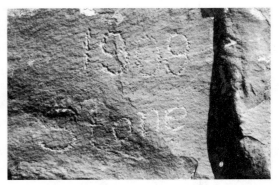

Julius Stone inscription, Ashley Falls. Marston Collection. *Reproduced by permission of The Huntington Library, San Marino, California.*

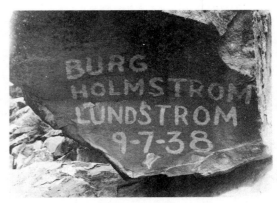

Burg, Holmstrom, Lundstrom inscription, Ashley Falls. Marston Collection. *Reproduced by permission of The Huntington Library, San Marino, California.*

Dellenbaugh was barely able to make out Ashley's inscription in 1871, and the last time anyone noted the inscription was in 1950, when peripatetic river runner Harry Aleson recorded finding it.[28]

The second important point about Ashley Falls that Nevills brings up is that it was actually a pretty easy rapid to run, despite the legends and dark stories of starvation and disaster. Even as Dellenbaugh labored to line

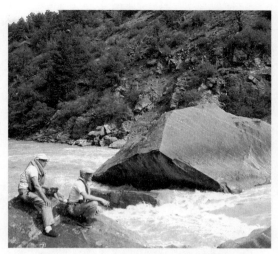
Fred Wood and Bob Parsons at Ashley Falls, 1955.

Powell's heavy wooden boats past the rapid in 1871, he was less than impressed, having been "brought up on Niagara."[29] By the time Norm Nevills got there in 1940, boats and techniques had advanced enough so that most river parties would run Ashley Falls, albeit usually only after careful study.

It was a tricky run at any water level. At low water, when most early expeditions went down the river, it was usually run on the right side of the huge central rock. Although there was no clear channel, a boatman could navigate a tight, difficult course through the rocks, usually knocking the boat against the boulders in a few places. The left side of the house-sized boulder in the middle was completely blocked at low water. At higher water levels, the right-side channel became difficult because of lateral waves that came at odd angles, almost ensuring a capsize if they were not entered just right. The left run, the preferred one at high

water, was made difficult by a huge standing wave that would inevitably fill a boat with water. There were exceptions to this; Les Jones ran the *Brontosaur*, a 33-foot inflatable pontoon, down the right side at high water in 1956 during the Eggert–Hatch Expedition and somehow made it through a channel barely wide enough for the boat without wrapping the ungainly craft around the big rock. Similarly, Al Morton and A. K. Reynolds ran their wooden cataract boats through the right channel at high water in 1950, because that was a better vantage for Morton's film camera. In the footage, both of them drift sideways and can be seen very nearly capsizing in the big lateral waves. But these were exceptions, and most river travelers ran right at low water, left at high water.

But for all the waves and holes and the huge "cubeular" rocks, the rapid could be run. Even if the boat filled with water or someone fell out, just below Ashley Falls was an enormous calm pool, without another rapid for over a mile. In fact, as Buzz Holmstrom noted in 1937, below was a shallow ford, with a trail crossing the river, where cattle ranchers often moved their herds from one side of the canyon to the other. Even when Ashley Falls was becoming familiar, though, it could still be dangerous, as Bill Purdy, who had been through Red Canyon "dozens of times," probably more than anyone else ever did, found out once in 1955:

Once in my foldboat I was alone and I looked at that rapid and I couldn't see why—the river was really high—and I couldn't see why I couldn't go right down the middle, right into the middle of the big rock and make a right hand turn because as you watched the water that's what the water did and I thought it would just take me right around. And so I tried it but it was a very bad mistake because I slammed right into the rock and it pinned me up against it and for a minute it was pretty exciting, but I managed to get out of it.[30]

One of the few who actually capsized a boat in Ashley Falls was Don Harris, by 1940 a seasoned boatman and veteran of Cataract and Grand Canyons. For some reason Harris, who was an excellent oarsman, always had trouble in Ashley Falls. In a 1990 interview he was asked if he had ever capsized a boat:

First time is when were on a USGS trip in high water in Ashley Falls and we capsized there. Pilot error, let's see had I known just exactly how the rapid was I should have pulled ashore. We ran down the left side of that big rock. If I could have had one of the fellows stand on shore and keep tossing some pebbles over where I was supposed to hit the break off then I'd have been in position. I was just about a boat width too far one way or the other, too far left I believe. If I would have been another boat width over I would have run it without capsizing.[31]

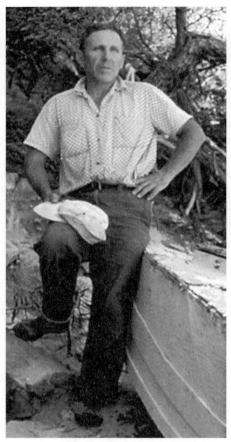

Don Harris.

Harris also wrote about the experience in a report to the Water Resources Branch of the U.S. Geological Survey:

During this high-water trip [June 1947], one of the boats was capsized in running Ashley Falls rapid on the Green River, but was recaptured several hours later, 19 miles downstream. Three boat oars were the principal loss in this accident, in

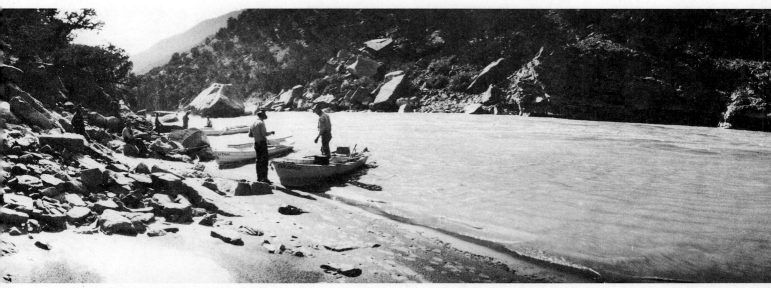

Pool below Ashley Falls, 1922.

addition to one day's time while extra oars were being rushed from Salt Lake City via Rock Springs, Wyoming, to the Browns Park area.[32]

So all of the worry about Ashley Falls by early river runners was actually for nothing. Cal Giddings, a pioneer Utah kayaker, ran Ashley Falls in the late 1950s and summed it up: "I remember we worried a lot about that because we'd heard about it, but it was pretty simple when we got there. So I think that was a little bit over-exaggerated in difficulty."[33]

Indeed, one of the ironies of this stretch of river is that all early river parties commented on how worried they were about Ashley Falls until they got there and discovered that it wasn't that bad. Then, relieved and incautious, they would go downriver about twenty miles and wreck their boats in Red Creek Rapid, just above the flat water of Browns Park. Red Creek was, and still is, a very difficult rapid that has been the scene of a number of wrecks and at least one death. Our story now returns to that rapid and the rest of Red Canyon.

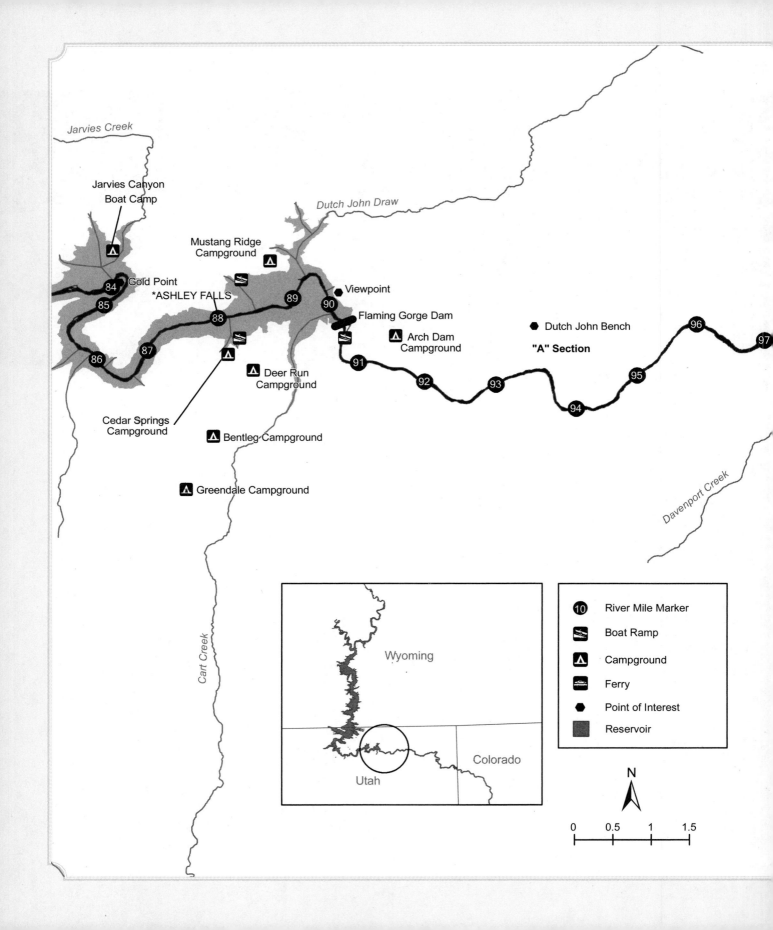

Jarvies Creek

Jarvies Canyon
Boat Camp

Dutch John Draw

Mustang Ridge
Campground

Gold Point
84
*ASHLEY FALLS
85
89
Viewpoint
90
Flaming Gorge Dam
88
Arch Dam
Campground
87
Dutch John Bench
86
"A" Section
91
Deer Run
Campground
96
97
Cedar Springs
Campground
92
95
93
94
Bentleg Campground

Davenport Creek

Greendale Campground

Cart Creek

Wyoming

Colorado

Utah

Legend

10   River Mile Marker

   Boat Ramp

△   Campground

   Ferry

⬢   Point of Interest

   Reservoir

N

0   0.5   1   1.5

THE REST OF RED CANYON

Flaming Gorge and its kindred canyons tell the tale of the centuries—the ever present story of Nature's struggle against Nature—the epic of water versus earth—the relentless attack of the elements upon the well-nigh everlasting rocks of the hills. The story is told in picture and in sculpture, and it is put to the music of the ever present roar of the mighty Green. Wild as the country is, it is the contrast which makes it wonderful. Calm waters, then the rush and the drag of the canyons, with the narrow stream tumbling and grumbling down across the hundreds of rocks which speck the bottoms. Then suddenly the canyon walls seem to sicken of the contest against the tireless river and they retreat to leave the river wandering around a meadow as if looking for someone to pick up the fight. Then as if the hells had renewed courage they again come to the river and the battle is on once more . . . Red Canyon came in the afternoon, and with it deer by the hundreds, and then a night camp at Skull Creek flats, where the stars seemed about to pop out of the skies and smite us for trespassing on their sacred soil.

—Russell Frazier (n.d.)

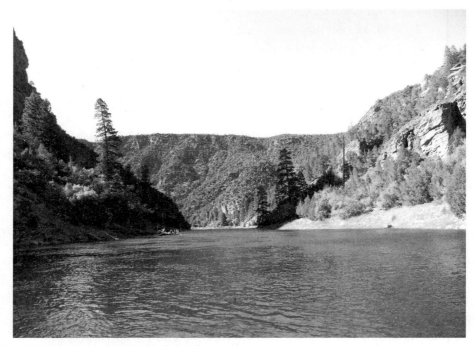
Red Canyon, just below Flaming Gorge Dam.

A lot of Red Canyon lies below Ashley Falls, with a number of smaller, unnamed rapids, such as the ones at the mouth of Dutch John Draw and Cart Creek. The draw was named for "Dutch John" Honselena, a German immigrant from Schleswig-Holstein who had such a thick accent that he was barely intelligible.[1] German speakers were often lumped together as "Dutch" during this time. Honselena had a small ranch headquartered at the mouth of Dutch John Draw, where the Green bent sharply to the south, but his corrals and fields were on the flat top of the canyon to the north of the river, which became known as Dutch John Flat. Dutch John had some mineral claims near Red Creek but mostly raised and traded horses for a living. Like many other small ranchers in the area, he often traded worn-out mounts for fresh ones with anyone who happened to come to his remote ranch, no questions asked—no doubt some of his patrons were outlaws.[2]

Cart Creek is a practical, typically rural name. Logging has also long been a mainstay of the economy around the Green through the Uintas, and the name comes from the big-wheeled carts used to haul logs. The mouth of Cart Creek was within sight of the location of Flaming Gorge Dam (but more of that

later). Many early river runners remarked that the stretch from Ashley Falls to Browns Park was the roughest part of Red Canyon: almost one continuous rapid, especially at high water. Jack Hillers, a member of Powell's 1871 crew—and himself a German immigrant and veteran of the Civil War—described this stretch and commented wryly on Powell's authority at the same time:

> The Major tells us we will have smooth water until we reach Ladore.
>
> June 6. Started out this morning anticipating smooth water but had not gone far when we heard a noise resembling a rappid [sic], but of course having been told that we would have smooth water, we thought nothing of it. But all of a sudden turning an angle we found that little rapid round the corner, but got through it all right. Down the river we went meeting rappids after rappids, some them as swift as 15 miles an hour. At dinner some one of the boys asked the Major if we would have any more smooth water, when he answered "well about the same" . . . After dinner ran some 10 miles of "about the same" as we had in the forenoon when all of a sudden we opened out into a beautiful

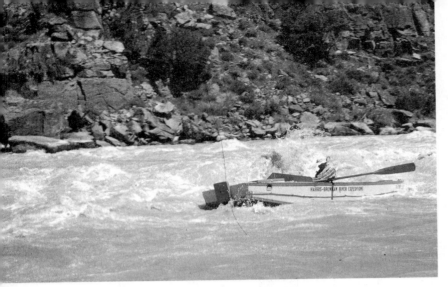

Red Canyon Rapids. *Collection of Roy Webb.*

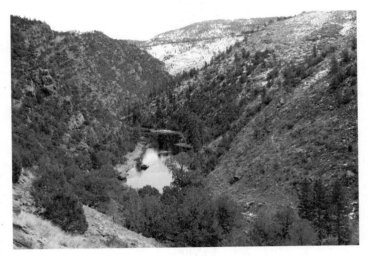

Red Canyon.

park. Major called it Red Canyon Park. We camped on right bank under two large pine trees.[3]

William Richmond—who was trying to chivvy a makeshift raft called *Tom and Jerry* down the river in 1896 loaded with prospecting equipment along with his partner, Frank Leland—would have agreed with Hillers:

From there on to Brown's Park we had many laughable experiences. The river became rougher with all kinds of rocks. *Tom and Jerry* became almost unmanageable, cutting all kinds of antics, sometimes going to one side of a boulder while our good old boat, *Nellie Gray*, with the whole family, including our dog, on the opposite side. And sometimes where the boulder happened to be too large for the rope to go around, she would leave the water and come dashing over the top of the rock and take a dive immediately behind the boat, much to Frank's discomfiture who would face about cursing and tell them to follow the boat which did not seem to do much good.[4]

Shortly after this, they met Nathaniel Galloway in Browns Park, who asked if they wanted to accompany him all the way down the river through the Grand Canyon. For Leland, however, Red Canyon had been quite enough; he and Richmond parted ways. Leland hiked out with their dog, while Richmond did go all the way down the river with Galloway.

But the rapids ceased for a while in Little Hole. Powell's Red Canyon Park later became Little Browns Hole, soon shortened to Little Hole. The river at Little Hole was shallow enough to be forded when the water was low, and a trail crossed the river there:

At that time, there were no permanent residents on the east side of the river in

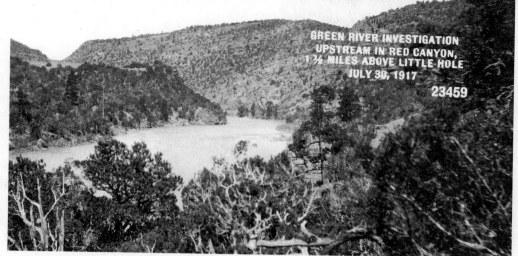

Red Canyon, just above Little Hole.

Utah. Stockmen grazed their stock on Dutch John Flat and Antelope Flat in the summertime, but the rest of the time this area was completely uninhabited. A trail down Little Hole was used in the wintertime by ranchers to get from Little Hole through Dutch John Gap and down to the river at the mouth of Henry's Fork where they crossed the ice on the river and then rode on to Manila to get mail and supplies.[5]

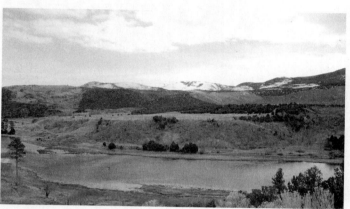

Little Hole.

Little Hole is the first large opening in the narrow confines of Red Canyon. Around 1885 Tom Davenport started running sheep in Little Hole. Davenport Creek is named for him, but one of its first full-time residents was Albert "Speck" Williams (sometimes given as Welhouse), an African American semihermit. Williams, whose mother had been a slave, was born shortly after the Civil War but by the 1890s had made his way to Rock Springs, Wyoming, and from there to Browns Park. There he made friends with Butch Cassidy and all the other outlaws. Williams suffered from a skin condition that caused large dark freckled patches on his skin and was universally known as the "speckled nigger." Perhaps because of this, and because it was difficult for African Americans in general during this time, he kept mostly to himself, living in various shacks and hovels up and down the Green River besides Little Hole. He also operated John Jarvie's ferry at the upper end of Browns Park for many years.

After the turn of the twentieth century Williams settled in Little Hole, where Davenport

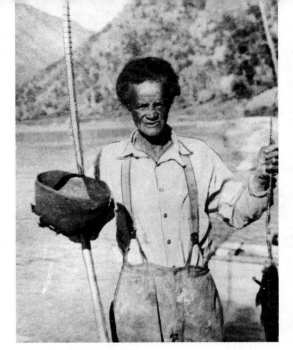
Albert "Speck" Williams.

Creek enters the Green. There he grew a few vegetables, fished, visited with people crossing the river on the trail there, and in general kept to himself. He told one friend: "If a black man wanted to survive in the West, he had to do good work and keep his mouth shut tight!" One job Williams excelled at was running a still. After Prohibition was passed in 1920, he kept thirsty residents well supplied.[6]

By the 1930s Little Hole was mostly empty, except for herds of sheep, until Orsen Burton bought the land (and the still) in 1942. Burton originally started a ranch near what is now Greendale, on the south side of the river in the open glades above the canyon, but he had long had his eye on Little Hole. Norm Nevills recorded meeting him there in 1940 and again in 1947; but after 1942 Burton planted alfalfa and an orchard and built a ranch house, workshops, and corrals just south of the river.

Burton sometimes financed his operations by rounding up wild horses on Dutch John Flat and herding them to sell in Vernal; if the snows were deep he would sometimes drive them far to the east, into Colorado, and back to Vernal. Horses and cattle were not his only source of income, however; he kept the still inherited with the property going for many years. When thirsty patrons found a number of dead insects in the bottles of moonshine that they obtained from Burton, "they did not despair. They just pulled out their handkerchiefs, strained the liquid, removed the bugs, and tipped the bottle. Perhaps this is why moonshine is sometimes referred to as 'bug juice.'"[7]

By 1955 the Burton family had put a great deal of work into the ranch at Little Hole, as noted by Marjorie Steurt, a passenger on river trip with Harry Aleson:

> A bulldozer put two ridges of rocks across the river, probably for irrigation water somewhere . . . We are coming to a ranch on the right. Green fields and three big hay racks. This is on low land just before we enter another section of Red Canyon. Cattle are racing along both banks. They are scared of us and since they are going down river, of course we are following them. Suddenly the sun has come out and there is blue sky filled with great fleecy white clouds. How good it feels.[8]

Just about two miles below Little Hole is another open area called Devils Hole, where

Jackson Creek enters the Green. Being so close to Browns Park, Devils Hole was also the lair of various outlaws and rustlers during the heyday of the Wild Bunch. Outlaw Billy Tittsworth reportedly murdered Charlie Powers there in a fight over some stolen cattle about 1885. Although Powers was buried by his friends, animals dug his body up from his shallow grave. Someone stuck his skull on a stake. No one knows the origin of the name "Devils Hole," but it perhaps came from the skull of the unfortunate Powers or the old cabins used as hideouts by outlaws, such as Butch Cassidy, Elzy Lay, David Lant, and Cleophas Dowd. In the 1920s the Boan brothers, Joe and Clarence, moved into one of the Devils Hole cabins. They had a few cows and some hogs and lived in somewhat unhygienic conditions, but mostly they made moonshine. One of the stills that Speck Williams tended was originally started by the Boan brothers.[9]

Even though the canyon walls were receding and Red Canyon was ending, travelers still encountered one obstacle before the calm waters and open vistas of Browns Park: Red Creek Rapid. Red Creek, which drains a large area of clay hills to the north called Clay Basin, not only gives the creek its color and name but is the source of frequent flash floods that have pushed big rocks into the channel. And Red Creek Rapid is a formidable one indeed, a long, narrow channel. The river is pressed up against a cliff on the right side and beset with boulders everywhere else. As if the rapid wasn't bad enough, along the banks were big patches of poison ivy. Red Creek seemed to sneak up on many early river travelers. After the buildup to Ashley Falls, and seeing that it wasn't all that bad, many would have a false sense that the worst was over and come to grief in Red Creek Rapid. It was first described in the early decades of the nineteenth century, by Thomas Jefferson Farnham, who was traveling west and passed through Browns Park:

> At seven in the morning we had breakfast and were on our way. We traveled three miles up the east bank of the [Green] river and came to a mountain through which it broke its way with a noise that indicated the fall to be great, and the channel to be a deep rugged chasm [Red Creek Rapid]. Near the place where it leaves the chasm, we turned to the right [north] and followed a deep rough gorge, the distance of five miles, and emerged into a plain [Clay Basin]. This gorge has been formed by the action of a tributary of the Green River upon the soft red sandstone the formed the precipices around.[10]

The earliest river runners—those who got that far—took one look at the long, rock-filled channel and lined around it as a matter of course. It was just one among many in lower Red Canyon, so they usually didn't say much about it in their journals and diaries. None of Powell's men mentioned it as such, because they lined most of the rapids anyway. But even someone who knew the river as well

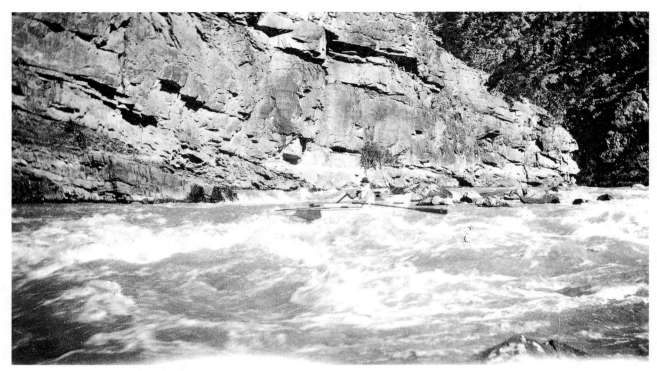

Red Creek Rapid, 1922.

as Nathaniel Galloway scouted it before running it. No one besides himself on the 1909 Galloway-Stone expedition had any river-running experience. He approached it with caution, as C. C. Sharp, who was also along on the trip, noted: "Red Creek is . . . a long, steep, shallow rapid with some waves about five feet high. Galloway considered this rapid difficult and we landed to walk along shore to select a course through."[11] After looking it over carefully, Galloway decided to let everyone else run their own boats through.[12] The Kolb brothers lined it two years later and went on; Bert Loper, head boatman for the USGS dam site survey in 1922, looked it over and then passed

through with no problems, but only after he "considered, very carefully, the work we had to do."[13]

But the next recorded travelers, the Todd-Page party in 1926, were not so lucky. Three young chums who had just graduated from Princeton—Web Todd, F. Lemoyne Page, and Ogden "Og" West—were seeking an adventure, so they decided to float the Green River. As a guide, they hired H. Elwyn Blake, who had been with Loper and the USGS party a few years before and had been a boatman on the Grand Canyon survey in 1923. Blake knew what he was doing, but Red Creek proved that even an experienced boatman can make

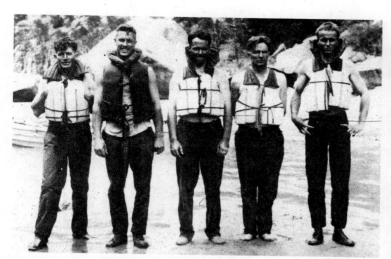

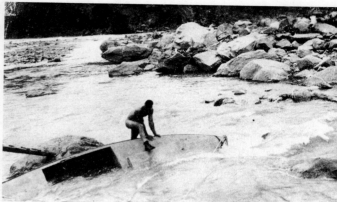

Todd-Page party, 1926 (left to right: Curley Hale, F. Lemoyne Page, Ogden West, H. Elwyn Blake, Web Todd).

Todd-Page party boat stuck in Red Creek Rapid, 1926. *Reproduced by permission of The Huntington Library, San Marino, California.*

a mistake. They reached Red Creek late in the afternoon of August 4 and wanted to camp just below, so Blake decided to line the boats past the first drop; this proved to be a costly error.

> All went well for a few minutes then suddenly the tremendous force of water caught the boat and threw her hard against a rock and before we knew what was happening she was tightly wedged between three rocks, and the water rushing hard against her . . . We all worked frantically for two solid hours until dark trying to get her off the rocks, but she stuck fast . . . No amount of prying, tugging, or pulling was of any avail.[14]

Most of the party's food and cooking gear was in the stranded boat, as well as the bedrolls and clothes of two of the men. After

herculean efforts, they were able to raise the hatches enough to get the soaked bedrolls out and spent a wet, cold night wondering what to do. Even a roaring fire and a bottle of "fresh raw moonshine" failed to warm them, so first thing in the morning they were up and at the problem. Some of them set to moving "several tons of rocks" in the channel to divert the flow away from the stranded craft. After hours of labor, the river was deflected enough to ease the pressure against the boat. Using driftwood logs, Blake then constructed a "Spanish windlass," a tripod of logs over the boat. They were able to tie a rope onto the boat and lift it straight up; with that and several other lines they were finally able to free it. Their other boat was still upstream, so Blake went up to run it through the new channel. He pushed off and jumped in, only to discover to his dismay that the oars were not in place, "contrary to river boatman's custom." As he was "fast approaching the channel which I least desired to enter," he grabbed the oars, hurriedly put them into their locks, and was just able to avoid running into the same rocks where the other boat had been pinned. Much sunburned and exhausted, they rowed into the quiet waters of Browns Park.[15]

It seemed as if no one got through Red Creek unscathed in those days. In 1936 Bus Hatch was stuck for almost three hours on a rock in the rapid before he was able to free his boat. In October of the next year, when Buzz Holmstrom was at the start of his solo journey along the length of the Green and Colorado Rivers, he took one look at Red Creek and decided to portage the rapid, the first time he had done so:

> [A]t 2:30 I came to Red Ck rapid—it is a dirty son of a gun to put it mild—steep long & rocky—at its head is a steep drop with water shooting into right cliff— a channel there but no room to use the right oar for the cliff—anyhow some lining had to be done below as the R[apid] splits into 3 parts. I might have tried to run it if close to home & everything favorable but there is too much to lose by a smashing—& portaging the boat over a beaver dam down a little side channel then run down a way with oars then slid over the rocks into another shallow channel & run down to the foot light—did not take over twenty minutes but then the trouble

began—it was over ¼ mile from the duffel at the head to the boat at the foot. I made it all in 3 loads but I am sure a donkey's ears would have burned with shame watching me—I got away from that place altho it was dark by the time I got the stuff in the boat—as there is just a long windy rock bar to camp on there—I hated to break down and portage as I have not done so before but what I am trying to do is to see how far I can get rather than how many I can run— If there are any more long portages, about half my stuff is going overboard.[16]

The next year, 1938, was significant in river-running history. Many elements of the past and future of river travel on the Green came together at one time. On the Green in the late summer and fall of 1938 was a wildlife survey from the Utah Fish and Game Department (one of the first such surveys along the river); a young man from Salt Lake City named Stewart Gardiner on a river trip in a new folding kayak (out for adventure); and Buzz Holmstrom (in the pinnacle of wooden boat technology) and Amos Burg (in the first inflatable rubber raft to float the waters of the Green). All of them made their way through Red Canyon, and Red Creek Rapid, with no real problems.[17]

Also on the river at the same time were the French kayakers: Bernard de Colmont; his new bride, Geneviève; and their friend Antoine de Seynes. Bernard, a filmmaker from Paris, had organized the expedition to film the "most wonderful river in the world," the Green and

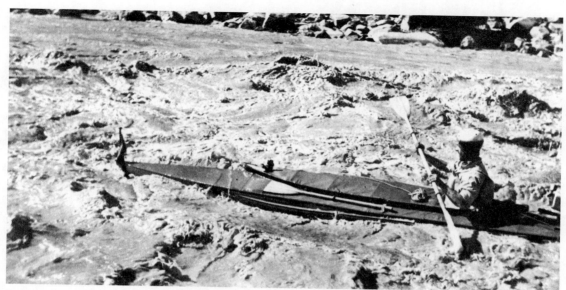
Bernard de Colmont in Red Creek Rapid, 1938.

Colorado. They came equipped with folding kayaks, oiled silk tents, Primus stoves, kayak helmets, a large supply of canned beer—they didn't trust the drinking water in the United States—and other gear that wouldn't be seen in America for another three decades. Departing from Green River in September, they made their way through the sandbars of the upper stretch of the Green, stopped at the Holmes Ranch to ride horses and play at being cowboys, and reached Ashley Falls about a week into their adventure. There Bernard ran all three kayaks through while Geneviève and Antoine filmed from shore. Bernard, already an experienced kayaker, was dismissive of the Green River and its rapids, as Antoine noted in his diary:

For a while we ask ourselves and we are surprised by the reputation this rapids

has. Bernard and Geneviève are always ready to minimize the difficulties mentioned by our predecessors and to consider them incompetent, over-fearful, big talkers, braggarts. This attitude is presumptuous and denigrating, *a priori*, it rubs me the wrong way and I have a hard time accepting it. But this time, I am ready to admit they are right.[18]

Antoine de Seynes's instinct that Red Canyon might not be as easy as they thought proved to be correct, as they learned at Red Creek Rapid. On September 21 they arrived at Red Creek—"the real thing this time"— and decided to portage their supplies. They lined two of the kayaks below the first drop, which turned out to be so difficult that Bernard ran the other one through. Then they repacked their boats and set out again, thinking that they were past the worst of the rocks. But almost as soon as they paddled away from shore, Antoine and Geneviève collided, causing Antoine to run onto a hidden rock; the current wrapped his wood-and-canvas kayak around the rock and splintered the wooden frame. Bernard and Geneviève were downstream by the time he extricated himself from his wrecked boat and were unable to cross the swift current to get to him.

> After exhausting efforts, I finally manage to free my broken boat, and take off behind it half swimming, half bounding down the rocks. I land at last on the left bank at the little beach where the Colmonts stopped. We unload and empty the boat a little, but with the right bank looking like a better place to camp, I have to get back in the water to cross. This prospect isn't inviting. I am shivering and exhausted. But I leave, pushing my kayak in front of me . . . On the right bank, we set up camp and I go to look for wood to repair the frame that Bernard is taking apart.[19]

While the French kayakers were working on repairing their boat, the Utah Fish and Wildlife Survey party led by biologist Lee Kay ran through Red Creek and pulled over to talk. The French kayakers, who had been warned about needing a permit to run the river, thought that they were about to be arrested; the Lee Kay

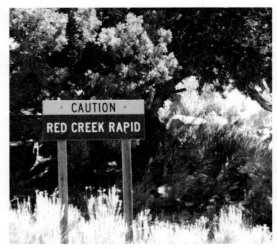

Sign for Red Creek Rapid.

party thought that they had been mistaken for outlaws. So the first meeting was rather cool. The misunderstanding was soon cleared up, however; the two parties ran the rest of the river down to Jensen, Utah, together, and parted good friends.

Norm Nevills ran Red Creek twice in the 1940s, as did a number of other river runners such as Don Harris, Bus Hatch, Frank Wright and Jim Rigg of Mexican Hat Expeditions, and A. K. Reynolds. All of them were in wooden boats, and in a rocky rapid like Red Creek too many hard knocks could spell real trouble. Immediately after World War II river runners began to use surplus inflatable rafts, which slithered and slid over the rocks and generally were much more forgiving in a rocky, narrow channel. But Red Creek could still be daunting, even in a rubber boat. Helen Kendall, on a river trip with Georgie White, the famous "Woman of the River" in 1959, recorded a run of Red Creek in a triple rig, an awkward craft made from three ten-person inflatable rafts tied side by side:

Georgie removed the motor and packed it safely away. Everything tied down. Life preservers put on and adjusted tightly, then, with Georgie and John on the left and Ringold and Eunice on the right, they rowed across the river to the right side where they stopped for final instructions while some of the men were on shore holding the boats, then jumped back on and rowed out from shore and we were on our way. Slid down the current and between two rocks, then between two more rocks about 14 feet apart and our boats were 17 feet. The bows slid up onto the rocks on the right and the stern, a corner of it, against the rock on the left. Slid between some rocks and around others, sat on one rock until John pushed us off. Sure looked like we were going to stay on that rock for a while. Slid over more rocks, turned around several times as we bounce against more rocks. Not a dangerous ride, but we got plenty of action while George and John were on the left oar and Eunice and Ring on the right. Georgie tried to give order which couldn't be obeyed in time, but we reached the bottom of the rapids successfully.[20]

Red Canyon ends in the calm waters of Browns Park only a few miles below Red Creek.

There are no more rapids, only a ledge of rocks pushed into the river to fill a ditch that used to supply water to the Jarvie Ranch, the first habitation in Browns Park below Red Canyon. Indian Crossing, an ancient ford about four miles below Red Creek Rapid, had been used by Indians for centuries and was later used by trappers, outlaws, and cattle ranchers. John Jarvie came from Scotland in 1880 and settled just downstream from the ford. At first he and his wife, Nellie, lived in a dugout, but later he built a stone house and store. Jarvie was an industrious man, well-educated and musical. He got along well with all of the other residents of Browns Park, whether they were miners, outlaws, or ranchers. His ranch became a center for the small society in the western end of Browns Park. Jarvie liked to write and recite poetry, play his organ and concertina, and entertain friends.

Over time Jarvie developed the ranch into a thriving outpost, with an orchard, vegetable garden, and cornfields as well as corrals, a blacksmith shop, a chicken coop, and other outbuildings made from railroad ties that had broken loose in Green River then been lassoed by cowboys and dragged from the river. Jarvie designed and built a large waterwheel to lift water from the river into a long ditch that irrigated fields just below the ranch and built a ferry to get across the river, which was operated by "Speck" Williams. Jarvie was a postmaster for that end of Browns Park and had a still where he made good whiskey. Alas, the outlaw legacy of Browns Park struck the Jarvie

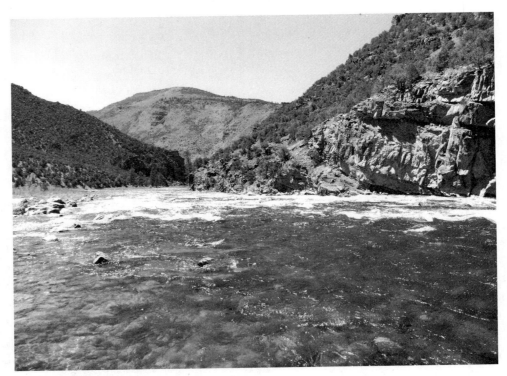

Red Creek Rapid today.

Ranch in a tragic way in 1909, when two criminals from Rock Springs robbed the store and murdered poor John Jarvie. They put his body into a skiff and pushed it off into the river, where it was found some days later near the Gates of Lodore. The murderers were never caught.[21]

The Jarvie Ranch has been restored as a historic site by the Bureau of Land Management; today visitors can go into the dugout, visit the store and the house, tour the grounds, and even visit the tiny cemetery where Theodore Hook and Jesse Ewing are buried. At the end of Jarvie's meadow is the Taylor Flats Bridge, a low, single-lane bridge left over from a planned 1960s development on the south side of the valley across from the Jarvie Ranch. The Flaming Gorge Recreation Company sold unimproved lots for as little as $299, advertising the area as "an outdoor paradise for hunters and fishermen." But like many such land schemes, the developers promised more than they could deliver and went out of business before power and water lines could be laid. All that's left today is a gridwork of empty streets that were never paved.[22] Along the river on either side of the Jarvie Ranch Historic Site are developed campgrounds for campers and fishers.

The Jarvie Ranch is traditionally considered the end of Red Canyon and the beginning of Browns Park. Browns Park has a rich history, and many good books have been written about it. But that is a different tale that has been told well and often elsewhere. To finish our journey down the Green River, we must now go back upriver about fifteen miles, to a spot just below Ashley Falls. By the time Helen Kendall wrote of getting "plenty of action" in Red Creek Rapid in 1959, events had been set in motion that would change the Green River forever. At a place within sight of the mouth of Cart Creek, the Flaming Gorge Dam was already under construction, and the Green would never be the same.

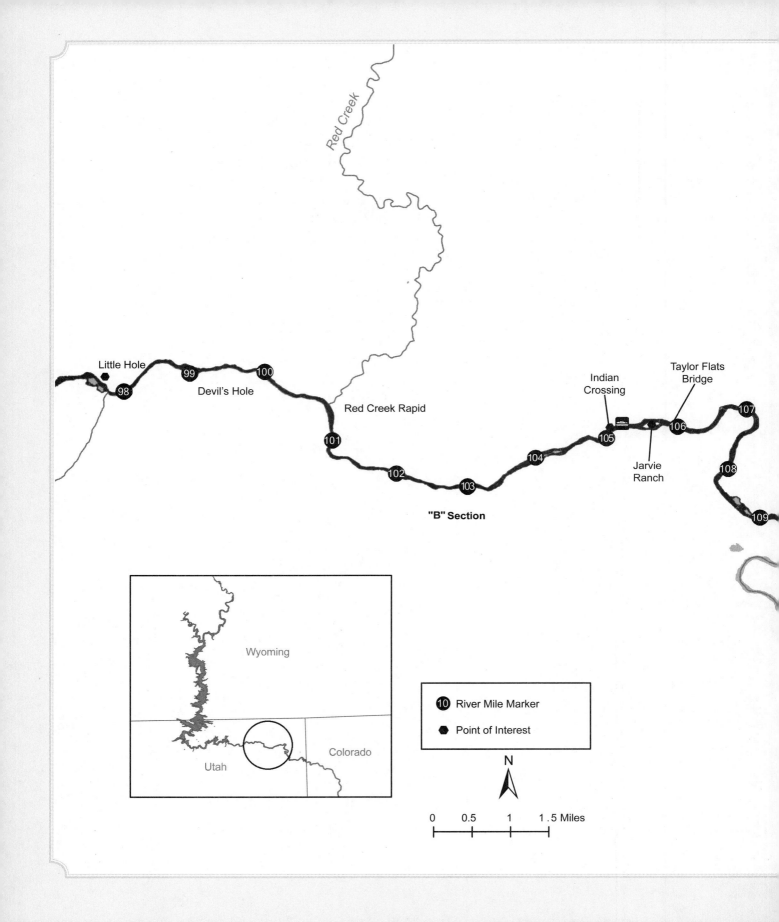

Red Creek

Little Hole
99
100
Devil's Hole
Red Creek Rapid
98
101
102
103
"B" Section
104
Indian
Crossing
Taylor Flats
Bridge
105
106
107
Jarvie
Ranch
108
109

Wyoming

Utah
Colorado

10 River Mile Marker

Point of Interest

N

0   0.5   1   1 . 5 Miles

THE DAM

The axis of Flaming Gorge Dam is very close to an old deer trail which the deer used in their annual fall and spring migrations from the high country down to the winter range and back again in the spring. The steep draw just below the outlet of the diversion tunnel was along the main trail. All the time we were working there, especially late November, there was a constant string of deer wading the river, even within 200 yards of the drill, on their way to Dutch John Bench and the area where they had spent the winter for many years. The present fence which surrounds the switchyard on the right abutment of Flaming Gorge Dam straddles this old trail. During recent years after the dam was built, the deer were forced to go farther downstream to cross the river, but hundreds of deer still winter in the pinons and cedars south of the town of Dutch John and on Dutch John Flat.

—J. Neil Murdock (1971)

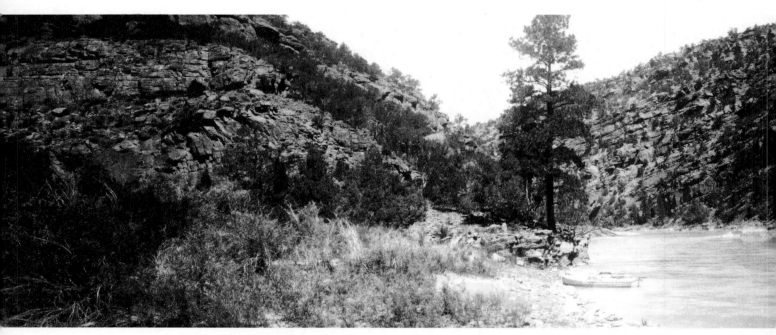
Flaming Gorge dam site, 1922.

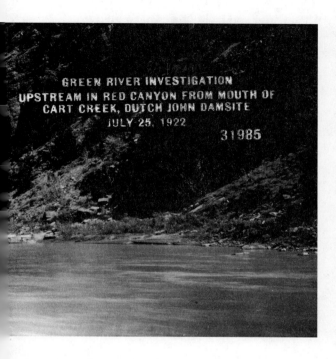

GREEN RIVER INVESTIGATION
UPSTREAM IN RED CANYON FROM MOUTH OF
CART CREEK, DUTCH JOHN DAMSITE
JULY 25, 1922
31985

Early Explorations

The Colorado River Storage Project was one of the most ambitious public works projects ever conceived. Impoundments were planned for a number of places on the Green River and Colorado River as well as on many of their tributaries. The title of one book about the project was *The Colorado River: A Natural Menace Becomes a National Resource*.[1] Construction of the Flaming Gorge Dam, only one of a number of units in the project, began in 1956; but people had been thinking about dams along the

Green River for at least fifty years before that. The U.S. Reclamation Service, the predecessor of the Bureau of Reclamation, recommended a dam in Horseshoe Canyon as early as 1904.[2] In the fall of 1909 Julius Stone and Nathaniel Galloway encountered a drill crew at the head of the Canyon of Lodore, some forty miles downstream from Red Canyon, trying to find bedrock for a possible dam; the crew had been there since 1907. In 1914 USGS hydrologist Eugene C. LaRue floated from Green River to Horseshoe Canyon in a "small, undecked steel skiff," along with an engineer from the U.S. Reclamation Service, inspecting potential places for dams.[3] Through the winter of 1914–15 crews drilled twenty-five holes in Horseshoe Canyon, but the Reclamation Service decided to try elsewhere. In 1917 Utah Power and Light sent a team overland along the Green. They hired a boat in Linwood and floated down to Hideout Flat, looking over the same sites in Horseshoe Canyon; but again, after more study, they decided against the site.

Things got serious in 1922, with the negotiations for the Colorado River Compact underway in Santa Fe, New Mexico. The Colorado River Compact forms the basis for all water rights between the states of the Upper Basin—Utah, Wyoming, Colorado, New Mexico, and

Nevada—and those of the Lower Basin, Arizona and, more importantly, California. As finally signed, the compact divides the water of the Colorado River equally between the two basins.[4] The USGS, in cooperation with various electrical utilities such as Southern California Edison and Utah Power and Light, organized river parties to survey the canyons of the San Juan; the Colorado in Cataract, Glen, and Grand Canyons; and the Green for prospective dam sites. The task of the Green River survey, under USGS engineer Kelly Trimble, was to identify potential dam sites, survey the side canyons up to the elevation of the maximum pool of the reservoir for each potential site, and make notes about the geology of the canyons, among other things. They left Green River, Wyoming, on July 13, 1922, after a dinner given in their honor by the Community Club of Green River, at which the locals regaled them with "vivid tales of unsuccessful attempts to navigate the canyons by daring adventurers."[5]

Besides Trimble and Woolley, the party consisted of J. B. Reeside, geologist; Bert Loper, head boatman; Leigh Lint and H. Elwyn Blake, boatmen and rodmen; and John Clogston, cook. Albert Loper by this time was a well-seasoned fifty-three years old; he had already spent years on the San Juan and in Cataract and Glen Canyons. There were no boating problems that he had not encountered and overcome before. While the newer boatmen got caught on rocks occasionally, Loper was always able to get them off. Once he was

upstream of Blake, whose boat was caught on a midstream rock. Loper steered his boat right at Blake's and knocked him free. The final member of the party—the one who portended the future—was H. L. Stoner, a representative of Utah Power and Light, a growing utility.

Their three boats were of the latest design: "Two of them were of the Galloway type, 18 feet long and about 4 ½ beam. The other one was 16 feet long and similar in plan to a common flat bottomed rowboat." The names were left up to the boatmen, who chose the three states they would traverse: *Utah*, *Wyoming*, and *Colorado*. Because earlier surveys had taken place, the real work did not begin until just above the mouth of Henry's Fork. After that the members of the party took their time, doing the first careful scientific survey of the valley and canyons of this stretch of the Green, plotting the elevation of a potential reservoir by hiking up the side canyons, taking geological samples, and making dozens of beautiful panorama photographs.[6] Along the way they met many of the people who had spent their lives along the river; little did any of them realize what this survey party foretold. They spent six weeks investigating the river from Green River, Wyoming, to Green River, Utah, making the first comprehensive topographic map of the Green in the process. Along the way they identified fourteen potential dam sites, including Echo Park Dam, at the head of Whirlpool Canyon, which would become the center of a national environmental battle; and the future site of the Flaming Gorge Dam.[7] Further survey work and

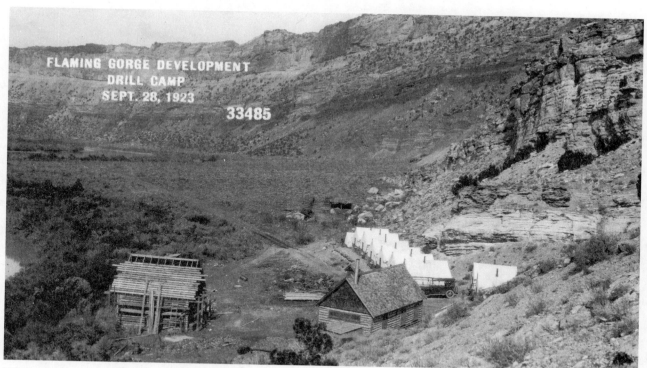

U.S. Bureau of Reclamation drill camp, 1923.

drilling of test holes went on through 1924, but the 1922 survey laid the groundwork for what would become the Flaming Gorge Dam.

Construction of Flaming Gorge Dam

Although the story of the Echo Park Dam controversy—one of the major environmental disputes of the twentieth century—has been told often and is outside the scope of this book, it does have a direct bearing on the construction of Flaming Gorge Dam. Suffice it to say that the Echo Dam was not built, despite the best efforts and fervent dreams of the Bureau of Reclamation; the congressional delegations of Utah, Wyoming, and Colorado; virtually all state and local governments in the tristate area; and numerous private citizens ranging from pro-dam groups who called themselves "Aqualantes" to churches and Chambers of Commerce. Repercussions from that decision swirl around eastern Utah and western Wyoming to this day, like eddies in a turbulent river.[8] One of the effects was to hasten planning and construction of the Flaming Gorge Dam.

The location of the Flaming Gorge Dam—in the middle of Red Canyon, just below the mouth of Cart Creek—had long been considered a good dam site. The solid, dense Uinta Mountain Quartzite provides a good foundation for a dam, and the northern latitude meant less evaporation than from reservoirs further downriver, in more arid, desert areas. A dam had always been planned there as part of the Colorado River Storage Project, but the defeat of the dam in Echo Park meant that the Flaming Gorge Dam suddenly had to be moved up on the schedule. The change caught Bureau of Reclamation planners by surprise. Some desultory preliminary work had been done there in the middle of World War II. Don Harris, who started running rivers on the lower Green and Colorado with Norm Nevills, still worked for the USGS and led river trips of engineers down the Green in 1944 and again in 1946. But they had been concentrating on the Echo Park Dam, so they had to switch gears quickly.

In the spring of 1948, as the Echo Park Dam controversy was beginning to heat up, a team from the USGS hired Bus Hatch to take them down the Green to Browns Park for another look at the sites that Trimble and Woolley had chosen two decades before.[9] Geologist Neil Murdock later wrote a history of the Flaming Gorge Dam:

> During the week of May 17, 1948, accompanied by engineers Hollis A. Hunt, C. H. Hard; Harold Chase, USGS; and Bus Hatch, boatman from Vernal, Utah, I made the trip from Hideout Canyon on the Green River to Browns Park. The purpose of this trip was the inventory and make a stadia profile of all the attractive damsites

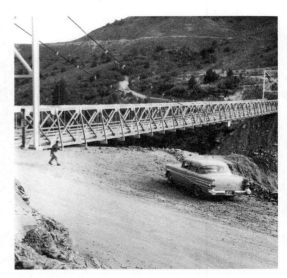

Temporary bridge near Cart Creek.

> between these two points. We used boats with watertight compartments which could run the rapids and if these boats became filled with water, they would not sink. Bus Hatch, who was familiar with all the rivers in this area and had gained quite a reputation as a fast-water boatman in these parts, was employed... The most attractive damsite found was at Mile 290 on the USGS rivers sheet and was a half-mile below the mouth of Cart Creek. This site was named Ashley Damsite after Ashley Falls which are located 2 miles upstream from the axis. The name was later changed to the Flaming Gorge damsite.[10]

As it became obvious that Flaming Gorge Dam was becoming a reality, more and more resources were devoted to the site. After President Dwight Eisenhower signed the enabling

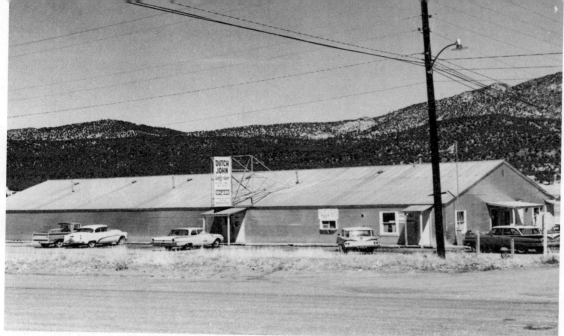

Dutch John, Utah.

legislation on April 11, 1956, work began in earnest. Arch Dam Constructors, a consortium of western construction companies, was given the contract and quickly got to work. Roads were bulldozed down to the site from both sides of the river so that workers and equipment could be brought in; and excavation of the keyways and the foundation of the dam began. A bridge was built over the river near Henry's Fork, and another just below Ashley Falls.

The workers improved older roads and set up camps on just about every flat place. Dutch John Flat was chosen as the site of a new town that would be the headquarters for the project and the dam after it was built, and workers, administrators, and families started moving into mobile homes there in 1957. Soon it was the largest town in Daggett County, with some 3,500 people living there during construction. It boasted a hospital, a post office, a service station, and a dining hall for the workers who lived in barracks.

Snowstorms, floods, and the remoteness of the location made the work harder, but it still went on. The hogbacks south of Linwood were found to contain gravel deposits that would be needed for the dam, and a crushing plant was built. Places that had only seen outlaws, Indians, and the occasional hermit or river runner and heard the roar of rapids and the call of wild geese now saw bulldozers, explosions, and surveyors and resounded to the noises of drilling, blasting, and mucking. A first step was to build a cofferdam, a temporary earth dam that would divert the river from its ancient bed into a diversion tunnel, to dewater the site so the foundation could be dug.

The diversion tunnel was over one thousand feet long and twenty-three feet in diameter, drilled through solid rock and lined with

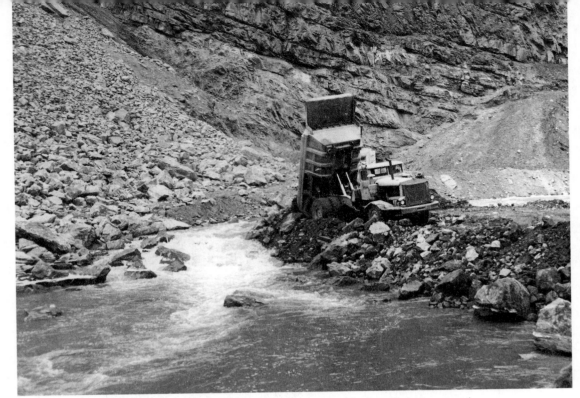

Building the coffer dam, 1956. *Used by permission, Utah State Historical Society. All rights reserved.*

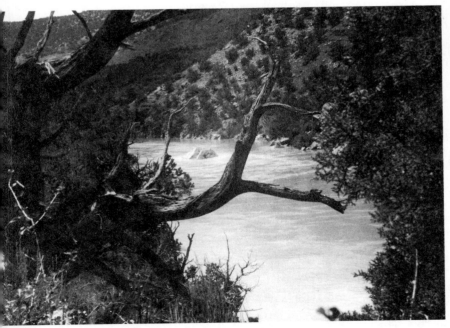

Ashley Falls partially flooded after the cofferdam was finished.

concrete. One of the first casualties of the construction was Ashley Falls, which was partially inundated by the water rising behind the cofferdam. The top of the huge, "cubelar" rock that gave the rapid its distinctive look could still be seen, but the historic river register was lost.

In 1957 the Green tried to reclaim the dam site; a huge flood of almost 25,000 cfs came down the river, but the coffer dam held, the diversion tunnel worked as designed, and the construction proceeded.[11] Site preparation was not finished until late 1960, but the huge pour of concrete started on September 18 of that year and only stopped when snow got so deep that the concrete trucks could not make it to the site. While this was going on,

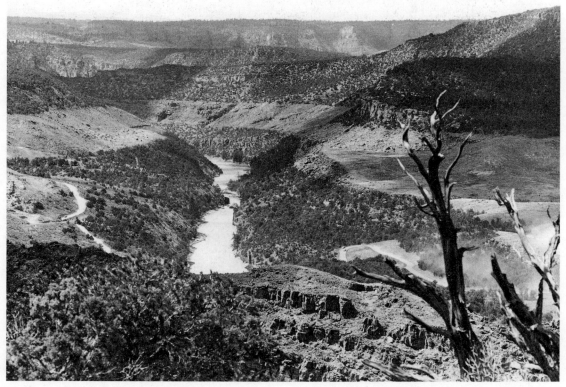

Timber salvage near Flaming Gorge Dam site.

other crews were sent out to salvage the thousands of board feet of prime timber that would otherwise be lost beneath the reservoir, giving the canyons a strange shaved look.[12] A sawmill was built next to the temporary bridge at Cart Creek to saw the logs into boards for transport. Burl Twitchell of Manila, who ran the sawmill, said that one ponderosa pine measured five feet across the stump and was almost one hundred feet tall. The trees upstream were rolled down the slope into the river and made into huge rafts, which could be floated down

to Cart Creek. This was still a dangerous job; one worker drowned when he fell through the log raft and was unable to get back up; his body was found below the dam site some days later.[13]

River Runners

Meanwhile people were still running the river. In fact, one similarity between Glen Canyon and Flaming Gorge is that after hearing about plans for both dams people flocked to the river to see what was to be flooded. Ted Hatch, a teenager at the time, remembered

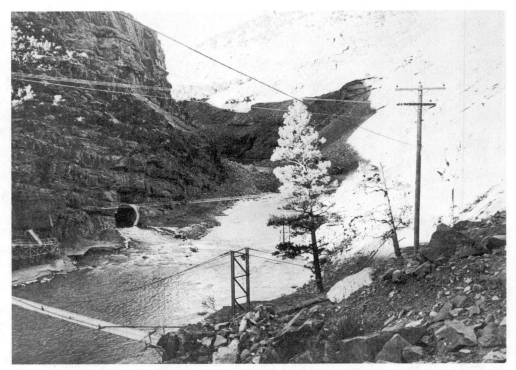

Flaming Gorge Dam site, 1958. *Used by permission, Uintah County Library Regional History Center. All rights reserved.*

that his father Bus Hatch booked charter trips for the Sierra Club, up to sixty people at a time. They would start at Hideout Flat and float from there all the way down the Green to Split Mountain, a seven-day trip. Ted would meet the party at the bridge at Cart Creek to resupply them with fresh food and later, after the dam site was closed to boating, to shuttle the boats and passengers around it.

By this time no one could escape the work on the dam. Mary Beckwith, on the 1956 Mexican Hat Expeditions trip, saw surveyors and a bulldozer right after running Ashley Falls: "A few miles below we heard the sound of

an automobile engine. . . . But it is only a bull dozer [*sic*] high on the cliff on the right bank; around the bend we surprise two surveyors on the left bank. No time is being lost in starting the Flaming Gorge Dam(n) site, it would seem."[14] Other boaters also ran into bulldozers, logging crews, and surveyors from Arch Dam Constructors. A. K. Reynolds continued to run trips down the river through the dam site, after checking with safety engineers and being given permission, as did Bus Hatch, Mexican Hat Expeditions, Georgie White, and Ken Sleight, who had just started his Wonderland Expeditions. A passenger on one of Georgie White's

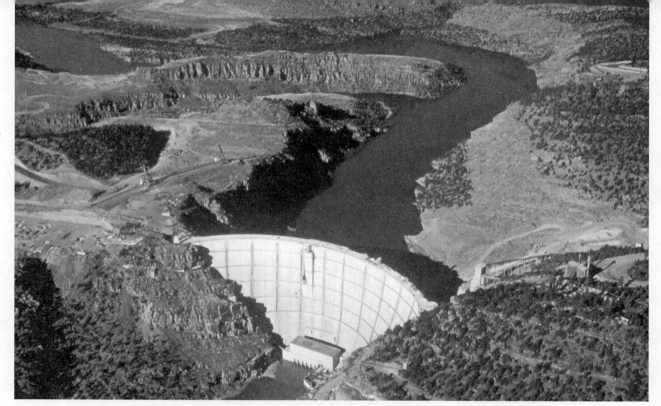
Flaming Gorge Dam.

trips in 1959 described the process of getting through the dam site while construction was going on. Whitey, Georgie's husband and driver, had already talked to the safety superintendent at the dam about allowing them to go through the site:

> Whitey was waiting for us [at the bridge just below Ashley Falls]. He had told us the day before that he had made arrangements with the safety superintendent for us to boat through the Flaming Gorge Dam site at noon. So we stalled around for more than an hour (the dam site was only a couple of miles downstream). We landed above the dam site about 11:15 am and I went looking for the safety superintendent.

Didn't find him but found lots of workmen who knew about us and told me he would wave us through at the appointed time. Sure enough at noon we saw a man in green clothes and a white hat waving a red flag at us. Since a red flag is usually a danger signal it took us a couple of minutes to decide he meant come on. When we caught up with him we stopped and talked for about 15 minutes. Many of the workmen were sitting along the river bank while they ate lunch. Most of them had cameras. They were taking pictures of us and we of them.[15]

But in June 1959 over 130 years of river travel on the Green came to an end, as noted in an article in *Desert Magazine*:

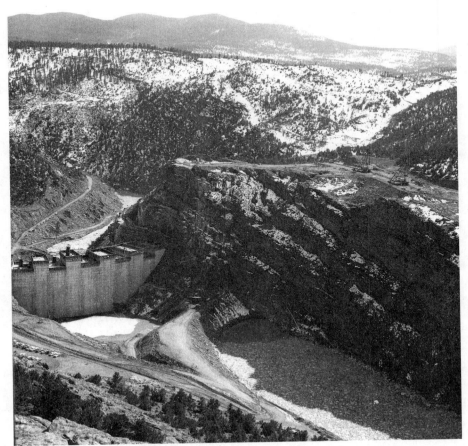

The dam rising (note the cofferdam holding back the frozen river). *Used by permission, Uintah County Library Regional History Center. All rights reserved.*

FLAMING GORGE DAMSITE CLOSED TO BOATS. The Bureau of Reclamation has closed the Flaming Gorge damsite construction zone to all boating. Officials said hazardous conditions on the Green River have been created by the blasting and scaling of rocks from the canyon walls at the damsite. Boating parties will be able to leave the Green River just below Ashley Falls at the new temporary suspension bridge built about two miles upstream from the damsite. From that point boats and gear can be transported by road to Little Hole and re-entry into the Green River . . . This summer a contractor is scheduled to clear the reservoir area in the 25-mile reach from the damsite to near Linwood, Utah. Boating in the canyon could be hazardous while the clearing operation goes on.[16]

Boaters were still allowed to get close to the dam site but had to leave the river at the temporary bridge just below Ashley Falls and truck their boats around to Little Hole. Typically, Ken Sleight was the last one to run a trip on the Green right up to the dam site and was one of the very few who actually raised a questioning voice about what was being flooded:

> During the latter part of October . . . we took our last river trip through Flaming Gorge and Red Canyon. A few days later water began backing up into the canyon reaches covering many important landmarks and historical markings including the Ashley and Galloway signatures. Rather than just get out at the Bridge crossing the Green . . . we floated right to the coffer dam (just above the diversion tunnel) at the now completed Flaming Gorge Dam. The water is now, at the writing 500 feet deep. We were the last party to make this run.[17]

Persistent rumors suggest that some river parties were allowed to run their boats through the diversion tunnel, but this hardly seems likely. Ted Hatch and a companion did drive a jeep through the tunnel once, just by acting as if they were supposed to be there.[18]

Salvage Surveys

At the same time, similar work was going on at the Glen Canyon Dam, far to the south on the Utah–Arizona border. In marked contrast

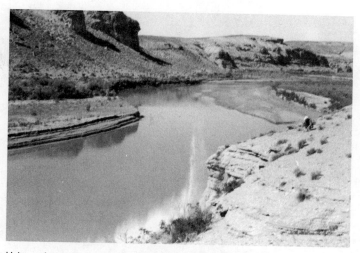

Using primacord to sample fish during salvage surveys.

to the Flaming Gorge Dam, however, large, well-funded survey crews from the University of Utah and the Museum of Northern Arizona were sent out to scour the banks of the Colorado and San Juan Rivers, documenting the thousands of archaeological and historic sites. Those surveys were carried on during the entire duration of the construction of Glen Canyon Dam and even afterward, as Lake Powell began to fill. Four volumes have been written on the results of the investigation into historical sites on the Colorado and San Juan Rivers alone, and many times that number about archaeological sites, vegetation, and wildlife. The Glen Canyon salvage surveys produced shelves of documents, thousands of photographs, hundreds of feet of color film, and vast collections of artifacts from archaeological excavations.

The same treatment was not afforded the basin of the Green River, soon to be inundated

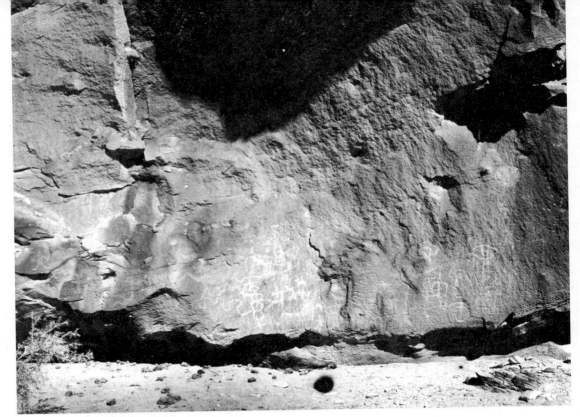
Fremont Indian petroglyph panel near Black's Fork.

by the reservoir behind Flaming Gorge Dam. The University of Utah was contracted by the Bureau of Reclamation to send out survey parties, two of which were led by biologists Seville Flowers and Angus Woodbury. During river trips lasting about a week they documented flora and fauna to be affected, recording vegetation along the river and within the reservoir pool and noting the different types of wildlife they encountered. They investigated the fish populations by detonating primacord in backwaters and eddies and collecting and identifying the stunned fish that rose to the surface.[19]

Most extensive, however, were the archaeological surveys carried out in 1958, 1959, 1960, and 1962. Some of the early fieldwork

was managed by Dee Ann Story, who was the director of the archaeology lab at the University of Utah and one of the first women to work alongside male archaeologists.[20] But the first preliminary survey was conducted in the summer of 1959 by William Purdy, whom we have met before. Purdy was not an archeologist but was familiar with the area. He was hired by Dr. Jesse Jennings, the head of the University of Utah's Anthropology Department and in charge of all of the salvage survey work in both Glen Canyon and Flaming Gorge. Jennings offered "$300 per month, $3 per diem, and $.07 per mile" if Purdy would use his own vehicle.[21] In a letter a month later, Jennings told Purdy to concentrate on the open country around the reservoir and not in the canyons themselves, noting: "I would expect very little in the gorge downstream from Sheep Creek."[22]

Jennings's instinct for the most part proved to be correct. Purdy talked to local residents such as Orsen Burton, Oscar Swett, and Sylvan Arrowsmith to see if they knew of any archaeological sites; it was their "unanimous opinion . . . that to their knowledge there exists not a single site in the canyon area that will be affected by the reservoir." The open areas above the canyons, however, were another matter. Dr. Jennings hoped to find evidence of Paleoindians, and Purdy's informants told him that there could even be a "pre-historic canal system." By himself, on unimproved roads, Purdy was only able to investigate a few easily accessible places such as the area around the mouth of Henry's Fork, where he found a large overhang near good water that he designated an archaeological site, noting: "If I were living in this country a thousand years ago this is where I would make my home."[23] Such romantic speculation did not stand up to the rigorous archaeological standards of Dr. Jennings, however, who reminded Purdy that "the subjective reaction of the surveyor to a site does not make it one. There must be significant evidence of aboriginal occupancy before we designate a site."[24]

Purdy spent the rest of the summer working on the archaeological survey of the areas that Dr. Jennings wished to investigate. But after that funds became tight, and he did not return after that first season in the field. In April

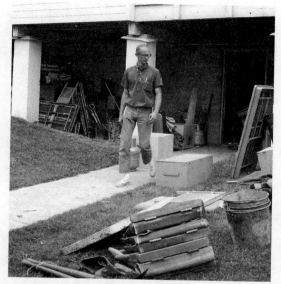

Kent Day, University of Utah archaeologist.

1959 Charlie Steen, regional archaeologist for the National Park Service, wrote to Jennings: "Whether we can do any more work at Flaming Gorge next year (either in archeology or history) depends on the appropriations."[25] Dr. Jennings was juggling two major projects at the same time. Glen Canyon was obviously much richer in archaeology and history, so he chose to put his limited resources there.

Some survey work was done in the Flaming Gorge area that year and the next by David Dibble; but the most work was done in the 1962 field season, under Kent Day. He and one assistant systematically investigated up one side of the reservoir pool area and down the other, concentrating on sand dunes and juniper-covered knolls, finding many likely temporary campsites, great concentrations of flint chips that showed where stone tools had

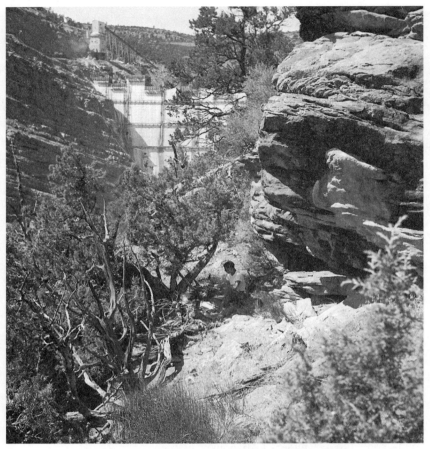

Prehistoric Fremont Indian site in Red Canyon with Flaming Gorge Dam in background.

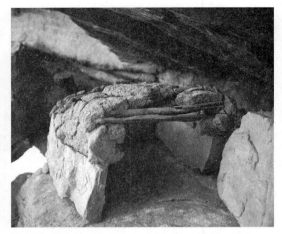

Prehistoric Fremont storage cist located inside alcove.

been made, and a number of petroglyph panels, including one near the mouth of Black's Fork that was "exceptionally large and complex" with "heavy concentrations of lithic materials." These panels showed standard Fremont elements such as bighorn sheep, geometric designs, and anthropomorphs (human figures). They also had some gray-ware pottery shards and a couple of small storage cists found in Red Canyon near the dam site. But

Day noted that he had seen a number of local "arrowhead" collections and in talking with residents had learned that such collecting was a standard pastime. This made him speculate that the area might once have had many more artifacts but that any surface sites had been picked clean. Even with that caveat, however, the area showed evidence only of temporary habitation. Day came to the conclusion that it was not worth putting any more time and money into the area. At the end of his summary report he revealed what were probably his true feelings about the value of the Flaming Gorge survey: "We are all eager to see some archeology to the south."[26]

It is unfortunate that those same resources were not devoted to the rich history of the area. In a document titled "Recommendations for Further Research," Dr. Jennings proposed an extensive program to document historic sites in the area: "The little town of Linwood should be the subject of a thirty day study on the ground. Recommended are extensive detailed photographs, measurements and architectural drawings of existing buildings. There should be an effort to construct, by means of a map, the original layout of the town showing all buildings which have ever stood in the settlement." He also suggested that "five days should be spent in photographing and recording architectural details of [the] Buckboard tavern," that research should be done in the National Archives in Washington, D.C., to look for photographs and documents that would shed light on the history of the town, and that the site of Ashley's first fur rendezvous and the 1872 diamond hoax should be sought.[27]

Notable by its absence is any interest in documenting the names recorded at Ashley Falls. It would not have mattered in any case, because none of this was carried out. In March 1959 Bill Purdy produced *An Outline of the History of the Flaming Gorge Area*, a 45-page document that covered the whole sweep of western history in the area to be flooded by Flaming Gorge Dam. Unfortunately, he spent a number of those few pages on subjects that were wholly outside the reservoir pool, such as Browns Park. The report contains only twelve black-and-white photos (and some of these likewise show scenes elsewhere), with only one general map. It includes no archival research, no extensive documentation of Linwood, the Buckboard Hotel, or the many cabins and ferries and ranch buildings that would soon be bulldozed and burned. Together these four documents published in the University

of Utah's Anthropological Papers series are under five hundred pages in length and contain fewer than one hundred black-and-white photographs.[28]

No smoking gun indicates why the Flaming Gorge area was given such short shrift in terms of salvage work. It is likely that the answer lies in the shortage of funding, however, combined with the obvious allure of the known archaeological and historical treasures to the south in Glen Canyon, along the Colorado and San Juan Rivers. Dr. Jennings only had so much funding and so many people to work in the field; Glen Canyon was where the archaeology was and, furthermore, where his students wanted to work. In the end even the Navajo Dam on the San Juan River and the Curecanti Dam on the Gunnison River got more attention and in-depth surveys than the Green River before their respective valleys were forever inundated.

The Human Cost

The construction of Flaming Gorge Dam also entailed a human cost. With the dam nearing completion, something had to be done about the many homes, ranches, corrals, and other buildings along the river; the Bureau of Reclamation did not want houses coming off their foundations and floating around in the reservoir (as had already happened with a few old log cabins), so they had to be relocated, dismantled and trucked away, or burned. All the years of hard work to build up the Holmes Ranch, the Brinegar Ranch, Keith Smith's "paradise" near Henry's Fork, the Buckboard

Hotel, Linwood with its octagonal dance hall and schoolhouse, and many other places on the river were for naught; those places would simply cease to exist. People from the Bureau of Land Management, which had been tasked with giving the residents the bad tidings, fanned out to tell the ranchers that they had to give up homes that some of them had lived in their entire lives. Many of the people who lived along the river refused to speak to any of the government employees. So the BLM promoted Alonzo Jarvie—who had been born and raised on Henry's Fork and was a grandson of John Jarvie of Browns Park—and charged him with persuading people to move out. The Holmes ranch, which had stood empty since Emma Holmes had moved to town a few years before, was one of the first to be burned and have its site cleared. On the Williams brothers ranch at the mouth of Henry's Fork, they "put up their last hay in 1958."[29] Many of the buildings from the Williams Ranch were moved to other locations all around the area; the old Finch house, which had been there when the family bought the ranch in 1930, was moved to Manila, as were some of the other homes. The garage, ice house, and granary were moved to Minnie's Gap, east of the reservoir. The property included two small family cemeteries, one belonging to the Finch family and one dating from the time of "Shade" Large. The locations of some graves were known, so the remains could thus be relocated. But others could not be found and were inundated when the reservoir rose.[30] They even transplanted trees from the property; a crabapple tree is now at Minnie's Gap, while a large pine tree planted by Keith Smith was moved to the Bureau of Reclamation headquarters in Dutch John. A similar diaspora of the people displaced from Linwood occurred; one of the Williams brothers moved to Manila, another to Pinedale, Wyoming, while other families moved to nearby communities or to Rock Springs and Green River, Wyoming. The tight-knit community around Henry's Fork and in Linwood was broken up by the rising waters of the reservoir.

The Brinegar Ranch house, built by William and Maddie Brinegar during World War I, was moved to the bluff overlooking the reservoir; the rest of the ranch buildings, corrals, shops, and pens were bulldozed into piles that were then burned.[31] William Brinegar's ferry built in Green River and floated down to his ranch was left where it was, still attached to its cable across the river. The Linwood school and some other houses in Linwood were moved to Manila, while others were trucked to local ranches such as the Currant Creek Ranch and the one at Minnie's Gap. Even the old trappers' cabins, some of the oldest buildings in the state, were not spared. Among them were cabins built in the nineteenth century by Baptiste Brown and Shade Large. These cabins were over a hundred years old even then. One of the few old cabins to be saved was Uncle Jack Robinson's, built sometime in the early years of the nineteenth century. Finding the cabin on the property when he bought it in 1900, Keith

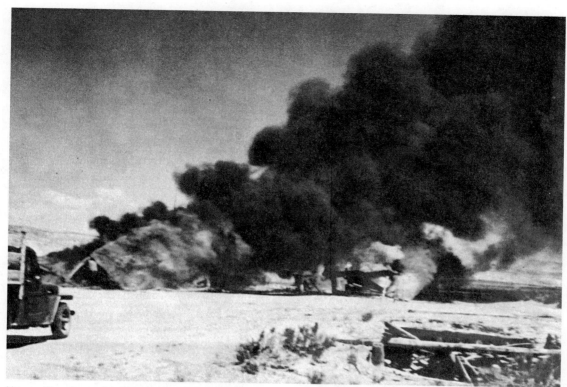

Linwood burning, 1960. *Courtesy Carol Lynn Gardner.*

Smith incorporated it into his house, where it served as the dining room. When Linwood was being razed, Smith moved the cabin to his new home called High Linwood in Greendale, just south of the dam, and attached it to the house in the same manner, where it still stands today.[32]

The most poignant story of the end of Linwood was that of George and Minnie Rasmussen. The town came down around them: all of the buildings that were not to be moved were bulldozed and burned in piles. In 1963 the contractor hired to clear the reservoir area, the Herman H. West Company, burned

down the Rasmussen Mercantile Store in Linwood, reportedly causing George to lose his will to live; he died shortly thereafter. Minnie, a tough frontier woman who was the daughter of Charlie Crouse of Browns Park fame, was alone in her home, the last building left standing. Minnie knew that she had to leave. Her only request was that they locate the grave of her father and move his remains, but despite a thorough search they were unable to locate the plot. When Alonzo Jarvie and the contractor in charge of moving or razing the buildings came to tell Minnie that she had to move, she invited them into her house for tea. During a congenial afternoon, they offered to move her house or any of her belongings; she said that she was still thinking about it. As Alonzo Jarvie drove home that night, he saw a cloud of smoke rising over Linwood and knew at once what had happened. Rather than let the BLM do it, Minnie had torched the house herself, belongings and all; she left the area that day and never returned.[33]

Opposition to Flaming Gorge Dam

Yet despite dramatic gestures like Minnie's and the enduring enmity of the many residents who were uprooted, virtually no real organized opposition to the building of the Flaming Gorge Dam arose. At the other end of Utah, where Glen Canyon Dam was rising, a chorus of voices already protested the loss of that wonderland; within two decades it would swell into an angry roar that still poisons relationships in Utah and Arizona. But that did not happen, and indeed has never happened, at Flaming Gorge. Instead, many people, still nursing their disappointments over the failure to build the Echo Park Dam, welcomed the Flaming Gorge Dam as a positive boon. The "Aqualantes" shifted their allegiance to the Flaming Gorge Dam and the reservoir soon to come, and local newspapers printed glowing editorials about the recreational opportunities and the jobs, water, and power that would begin to flow as soon as the dam was completed and the gates were closed. Even before completion, the dam provided jobs for hundreds of workers for years. The Sierra Club,

which had fought the Echo Park Dam so bitterly, backed out of the fight when it came to the Flaming Gorge Dam and even listed it as a tourist attraction in a brochure advertising river touring section trips: "At Ashley Falls Rapids, just above the damsite area, we take our boats out and shuttle about thirteen miles around construction. This will be an entirely different type of adventures, with an opportunity to see a major dam being built."[34]

This is not to say that no one opposed the construction of the dam. Besides Ken Sleight (mentioned above), another dissenting voice was that of Don Hatch, son of famed riverman Bus Hatch. Bus and Don had been opponents of the Echo Park Dam when it was a very unpopular stance in their home of Vernal, Utah. Don later talked about the loss of the upper canyons of the Green in an oral interview in 1984: "[T]he living space was the bottom of the canyon . . . where all the deer were—the animals, the geese and all of these; the wildlife was along the bottom. So when you put the dam there and flooded it, it essentially killed all the living space for animals. There were a lot of animals there . . . the beauty of the canyons seemed to be the bottomlands of the river—the immediate bottomlands . . . you take a picture of the canyon the way it was then— and it's a beautiful picture—and then if you take the scissors and cut off the bottom third, that's what it looks like now."[35]

But for the most part opposition to the Flaming Gorge dam, as opposed to the Glen Canyon Dam, was merely a whisper. Why were the communities and ranches along the river, as well as the scenic wonders and thrilling rapids of Flaming Gorge, Horseshoe, Kingfisher, and Red Canyons, allowed to be irrevocably altered without a single major note of disagreement? One reason has to be the fight over the Echo Park Dam. The forces that had gathered to oppose it were exhausted by the years it had taken to save Dinosaur National Monument from inundation; they had neither the heart nor the resources for another such struggle. Another factor was that environmental groups and others adamantly opposed to Echo Park Dam tacitly, or in some cases openly, offered up both the upper Green and Glen Canyon as alternatives for dam sites. Even David Brower, the head of the Sierra Club and the stalwart of the fight against the Echo Park Dam, suggested that Red Canyon was a better place for a dam than Echo Park.

That is another key factor: just like Glen Canyon, the valley of the upper Green River was not in a national park or monument or in a designated wilderness area. Neither place had any statutory protection that would provide a reason to save it, as being in Dinosaur National Monument did for Echo Park. Like Glen Canyon, the Green River region was a remote, all but inaccessible area (except for the people who lived there). It was little known outside Utah and Wyoming, with few visitors and no real constituency to rise up against its loss. The development of water resources for irrigation and storage had always been viewed in Utah

as almost a sacred trust, a religious necessity—"make the desert blossom as the rose," as the saying went. It was scarcely less so in more secular Wyoming. Finally, this was the era of the Red Scare and the missile gap, of McCarthyism and the Soviet menace; a line from a pamphlet produced by the Aqualantes favoring the Echo Park Dam could just as easily refer to the Flaming Gorge Dam: "Under the threat of atomic warfare, industries are scattering to the sparsely populated areas of the West. These industries need power in amounts that can come only from large-scale power dams."[36] Opposing the Flaming Gorge Dam would have been unpatriotic!

It would not have mattered anyway. Construction was proceeding at a rapid pace. The gates on the rising dam were closed on November 1, 1962, and the last bucket of concrete was poured two weeks later. The first generator had been installed in September, and President John F. Kennedy visited Salt Lake City to press a key and start the generator on September 27, 1963. Commercial generation of power began on November 11 of that year. This was one of Kennedy's last official acts; he was assassinated in Dallas a short time later. After more generators were added, President Lyndon B. Johnson and his wife, Lady Bird Johnson, dedicated the dam and reservoir on August 17, 1964. The dam had taken just over seven years to build, at a cost of $65,297,407. For their money, taxpayers got a thin-arch concrete dam 502 feet high, 1,285 feet across the top, and 151 feet wide at the

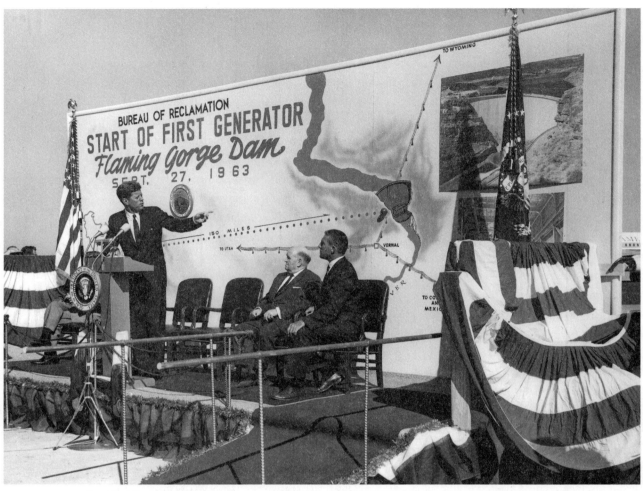

President Kennedy starting the first generator at Flaming Gorge Dam, September 27, 1963. *Used by permission, Utah State Historical Society. All rights reserved.*

base, containing almost a million cubic yards of concrete. It has three 52,000 horsepower generators that can produce 36,000 kilowatts each. At MPE (Maximum Pool Elevation) the reservoir backs up ninety-one miles, to within four miles of the town of Green River, Wyoming, and stores up to 3,789,000 acre-feet of water.

The Naming of the Reservoir

One minor controversy that did arise was about what to call the reservoir. The one on the Colorado, far downstream, was to be named for John Wesley Powell, but differences arose among historians, local residents, and politicians who had shepherded both dams through Congress about what to name its sister to the north. One surprising candidate emerged even before the dam was finished: a resolution passed by the Wyoming State Legislature calling for the reservoir to be named "Lake O'Mahoney" for Senator Joseph O'Mahoney of that state. This caught many by surprise, for Senator O'Mahoney was not a household name in Utah or even, in all probability, in Wyoming. He served on the Senate Committee on the Interior and had been influential behind the scenes in Congress, shepherding the dam through the approval and funding process. A compromise was proposed, whereby the Wyoming section of the reservoir would be named for the senator and the Utah portion for William Ashley, but this was deemed too confusing.[37]

Ken Sleight, ever the activist, penned a letter to the editor of the *Salt Lake Tribune* as soon as he heard the suggestion, saying: "NAME IT LAKE ASHLEY. It has been suggested that the lake formed by Flaming Gorge Dam in northeastern Utah be named for the late Senator O'Mahoney of Wyoming. This would indeed be a mistake." He went on to list six reasons why the lake should be named for William Ashley and followed up with letters to Utah senators Wallace Bennett and Frank Moss and Utah's governor, George Dewey Clyde. Senator Bennett agreed, telling Sleight that—despite his fondness for his distinguished colleague in the Senate—he would not go along with naming it for O'Mahoney.[38] Sleight then sent a letter to Otis Marston, who had set himself up as the historian and overall

clearinghouse for all information about the Colorado River: "Just recently Dock—there is a movement to name the lake behind Flaming Gorge O'Mahoney Lake. Forbid! As soon as I first heard of it—letters went flying to several congressional representatives, etc. I prefer the name Ashley Lake. If it is not named that—it should be retained as Flaming Gorge—even though Flaming Gorge Canyon accounts for only a small portion of the lake."[39]

After President Kennedy was assassinated in November 1963, Senator Frank Moss of Utah proposed naming it "Lake Kennedy," since one of the late president's final official acts had been dedicating the dam. A displaced resident of Linwood even proposed that the lake be named after that town.[40] But in the end the name "Flaming Gorge Reservoir" was officially adopted.

Downstream Effects

The drastic effects of the new dam and the rising reservoir were not confined to just the area above the dam, however. The Green, once muscular and muddy and seasonal, was tamed by the dam. In order to fill the reservoir quickly, engineers basically shut down the river, allowing only a trickle to escape. Downstream in the Canyon of Lodore, a group of hikers walked down the river, the first to do so since Joe Walker had led a group of trappers on horseback down the frozen river in the 1830s. In Green River, Utah, the river all but dried up, alarming local melon farmers, according to a contemporary newspaper article: "FLAMING

GORGE STORAGE PROJECT DRIES UP GREEN RIVER FARMS. A team representing irrigators in the Green River [Utah] area has gone to SLC to ask for a release of water from Flaming Gorge Dam in an effort to boost the Green River water level and save cropland there. Sagging stream flow of the Green River has left the river so low that valley irrigation canals have gone dry."[41]

The most marked effects, however, were on the native fish. The cold, clear water that was now being released from the dam had a devastating effect on the big fish that had thrived for untold millennia in the warm, muddy waters of the Green River. The razorback sucker, Colorado pikeminnow, humpback chub, and bonytail chub were not adapted to live in those kinds of conditions and began to die off. Their survival was further endangered when the Utah and Wyoming fish and game departments, "paving the way for trout," decided to rid the river of "trash fish" by pouring over 21,000 gallons of the fish poison rotenone into the main channel and into backwaters and sloughs. Despite objections from biologists and conservationists, the agencies went ahead with the plan in September 1962, even before the dam was completed. Hundreds of thousands of fish were killed and piled up in eddies and backwaters; they reeked for months all the way down the Green River.[42] The river was now safe for trout and soon became a blue-ribbon fly fishery—or was it safe? After about a decade biologists noticed that the trout populations were decreasing and that the remaining fish were not reproducing. Studies indicated that the water, which was drawn from hundreds of feet below the surface of the dam, was depleted of oxygen and so icy (barely 40 degrees Fahrenheit) that it was too cold even for trout. In order to protect the fishery, by now a major generator of revenue, shutters were built on top of the dam at a cost of some $5 million, which mixed warmer surface water with the water that flowed through the generators.[43] That seemed to improve the conditions enough so that the trout fishery returned and is once again a destination for fly fishers from all over the country.

The dam was completed, and the waters began to rise. Within a few years the reservoir behind the dam had become, if not a "playground for millions," at least a destination for thousands of visitors per year. Flaming Gorge National Recreation Area was designated on October 1, 1968, including a number of marinas, campgrounds, boat launch ramps, and facilities for storage and servicing of boats. Typically, National Recreation areas are managed by the National Park Service (NPS). But after a few years, in a heartening display of interagency cooperation, the NPS relinquished control of the Flaming Gorge National Recreation Area to the U.S. Forest Service, because the area is surrounded by the Ashley National Forest.[44] Places like Linwood, the Holmes ranch, and the Buckboard Hotel lent their names to bays and marinas on the reservoir. Today many people in Daggett County, Utah, and Sweetwater County, Wyoming, make their living serving visitors who come to Flaming Gorge Reservoir.

The Lucerne Marina—named for the Lucerne valley—is the largest on the lake. It can dock 185 boats and offers houseboat, ski boat, and fishing boat rentals as well as a number of developed campgrounds on the lake. Giant fish lurk in the deep waters of the reservoir, and many record-sized lunkers are pulled from the water each year. Just as the planners imagined, Flaming Gorge Dam has proven to be a bonanza for Sweetwater County in Wyoming and Daggett and Uintah Counties in Utah. The stunning scenery and blue-ribbon fishing draw tens of thousands of people to Flaming Gorge Reservoir and to the Green below the dam each year to boat, water-ski, fish, and camp. According to a recent article in the *Salt Lake Tribune*, "Utah officials say Flaming Gorge Reservoir and the Green River below it support nearly 540,000 angler hours each year with an estimated annual value to Utah and Wyoming economies of more than $15 million."[45]

One significant part of that revenue comes from the blue-ribbon fishery that has developed below Flaming Gorge Dam. At the time the dam was built, the Green was considered a general fishery, meaning that any means could be used to catch fish. There were few limits on how many fish or what sizes could be caught and kept. Whenever the local fish and wildlife service would plant trout in the river, people would flock there and quickly fish it out. As a result, some of the local residents sought a change in legal status from a general fishery to a special-use fishery, which is more heavily regulated. One of those was Russ Perry, a resident of Vernal, Utah, who had fished on the river for years but recognized that in order to protect the fishery something had to change.[46] Russ and like-minded anglers started a petition drive, asking the U.S. Forest Service to make the change. But it was fiercely opposed by some local anglers and the lodges who depended on their business. Those working for the change prevailed, however; in the 1980s the Green River below Flaming Gorge Dam was officially declared a "blue ribbon fishery," which limits the numbers and sizes of fish that can be kept once caught and imposes regulations on when fish can be taken and on other factors.

As noted above, at first the fishery suffered from the cold and oxygen-depleted water released from the dam. But after 1978, when the shutters that mixed warmer surface water with the cold outflow used to generate power were completed, the trout population began to increase.[47] After that, interest in the area skyrocketed and has shown no sign of decreasing. Local lodges and guide services, which had originally opposed the regulatory change, now advertise the wonderful fishing to be found below the dam. Today fishing below Flaming Gorge Dam draws avid anglers from all over the world, to the tune of three thousand guided trips down the Green per year. Just the fees for guided trips alone generate millions of dollars, and the other economic impact is immense.

Other types of trout, such as browns (*Salmo trutta morpha fario*) and rainbows (*Oncorhynchus mykiss*), have been introduced.[48] The brown trout in particular have become a self-sustaining population.

Income from fishing now exceeds income generated by the ski industry in some measures, and the fishery below Flaming Gorge Dam creates more revenue for the State of Utah and Daggett County than do boating and other activities on the reservoir itself. Over 100,000 travelers visit the stretch of the Green below the dam annually, with over 5,300 annual guided fishing trips that contribute almost $2 million to the local economy. It must be said that not all longtime anglers view this increase in interest in the stretch below the dam as a positive development; some say that they will no longer fish the Green below the dam because competition for a favorite fishing hole has gotten too fierce.[49]

Before Flaming Gorge Dam, all of the many rapids and riffles below Ashley Falls except Red Creek Rapid were nameless, just more of what Hillers called "rappids after rappids [*sic*]." The names like Deadman Rapid, Little Steamboat Rapid, and Mother-in-Law Rapid that appear in modern fishing maps and guidebooks came about after the stretch of the Green below the dam became so well used by fly fishers.[50]

Other conflicts have arisen as well. Now that the Green no longer runs in seasonal cycles of flood and drought, many more people than ever floated the Green in the days before the dam are now able to run the rapids of lower Red Canyon. These range from experienced fly-fishing guides in expensive drift boats leading well-heeled clients to church groups to great gaggles of Boy Scouts in rented boats. Boats and equipment can be rented at a number of lodges near the dam. The stretch from the dam to Little Hole, with an easy shuttle and many splashy rapids, is especially popular. No permits or levels of experience are needed for this kind of use. The U.S. Forest Service, which manages the river, requires the use of personal flotation devices and hopes for common sense. But regulatory agencies provide very little supervision below the launch ramp. Consequently, inexperience and inattention lead to numerous reported capsizes, wrapped and damaged boats, hypothermia from the frigid water, and even some drownings. The crystal-clear water released from the dam allows lost gear from these accidents to be seen lining the bottom of the river below each of the rapids, including coolers, fishing poles, chairs, and other camping equipment. A big rock sticking up out of the river at Little Steamboat Rapid, about a mile and a half below the dam, has proven to be an especially dangerous obstacle for the unwary and has been the scene of a number of wrapped boats and several deaths.

This recreational use has also become a source of contention between serious fishers and casual boaters. The fly-fishing industry is heavily regulated. Only ten outfitting services are allowed to guide clients for fishing, and they pay substantial fees and contribute greatly to management and protection of the resource in terms of funding and time and effort. Casual recreational users are essentially unregulated, as noted above. Aside from boat rental fees and gas from the local service stations, they provide little or nothing in the way of assistance for cleanup and maintenance of campgrounds or in working with regulating agencies that manage the river. One fly-fishing guide went so far as to say that the heavy recreation use is a deterrent to development of the fly fishery and that without this recreation pressure the Green River below Flaming Gorge Dam would be unmatched anywhere in the world for its scenery, wildlife, and fishing.[51]

These conflicts and problems could occur anywhere in the West as states have grown, population has increased, and more people need more resources—whether water or land or recreation or a favorite fishing hole. Michael Johnson, author of the Utah Statehood Centennial Series volume on Daggett County, summed up the impacts of the dam on the county and, by extension, on the Green River itself:

> [T]he verdict on the overall benefit of the Flaming Gorge project is still a matter of contention. Many [Daggett] county residents and thousands of boaters, water-skiers, and fishermen would give an enthusiastic "yes" if the question was put to them. However, some older county residents and a growing number of environmentalists would offer a resounding "no" in answer to the question. There is no consensus; there is only the reality that this tour de force in concrete and steel has irrevocably changed the course of Daggett County history.[52]

"Ah well," as Major Powell said, "we may conjecture many things."[53] The dam is now an immutable fact of life along the Green River and will probably continue to be so long after humankind has reduced itself to ashes and the rodents and insects are the masters of the world. The history of the upper Green River, including the ranches, Linwood, and Ashley Falls, lives on in photographs, films, and the memories of those who were there. At least some small stretch of Red Canyon can still be seen and enjoyed. For those parts that are now forever altered—the open country of ranches and badlands, the spectacular Flaming Gorge, charming Horseshoe and Kingfisher Canyon, Red Canyon with its rapids and pines—it is better to remember the canyons as they were: beneath the waters of the reservoir a river once flowed. Cal Giddings, a University of Utah chemistry professor who was also a pioneer kayaker, can speak for all of those who remember what it was like to run the lost canyons of the Green River:

> One characteristic of those canyons—those are probably the most ideal places for beginning river runners to get going. They were fairly big waves but easy and straightforward. It was very beautiful . . . We worried a lot about Ashley Falls

but it was pretty simple . . . a good part
of that area was forested . . . I remember
one morning having mist hanging over the
canyon, hanging over the forested walls; it
was one of the loveliest sights I've seen on
the river.[54]

As towns go, Linwood, Utah, on the Utah–Wyoming border in the far northeastern corner of the state, wasn't much. There were a couple of general stores, a dance hall, a school, a saloon, and some scattered homes at the end of a long dirt road, isolated from other towns in either Utah or Wyoming. Along Henry's Fork of the Green River, which ran through town, there were some ranches and farms, and not much else. *Utah: A Guide to the State*, the WPA guide published in 1941, gave it only a couple of sentences, calling it "a group of weathered log buildings," and noting that it had a population of 74.

But what it lacked in size, it made up for in history and community. Native Americans had thrived in the area around Henry's Fork since time immemorial: Paleoindians hunted along its banks, the mysterious Fremont left rock art nearby, and the Shoshone called it home for generations. In the 1820s, the first mountain man rendezvous was held nearby, and trappers recognized that it was a good place to live. After the town was established in the late nineteenth century, succeeding generations lived, worked, and were buried in Linwood; couples were married, babies were born, and a close-knit community grew up. All of that changed in the 1950s, when forces far distant from the tiny hamlet were set in motion that would result in the town's obliteration. Linwood was not even allowed the genteel slide into being a ghost town; instead, to meet the demands of the Bureau of Reclamation, Linwood and the ranches along the river were uprooted and moved, or bulldozed and burned. Now Linwood is just a name on the recreation maps of Flaming Gorge Reservoir, and the site of the town is under a hundred feet of cold water. But the community of Linwood survives in the fond memories of the people who grew up there and in the photographs found on these pages.

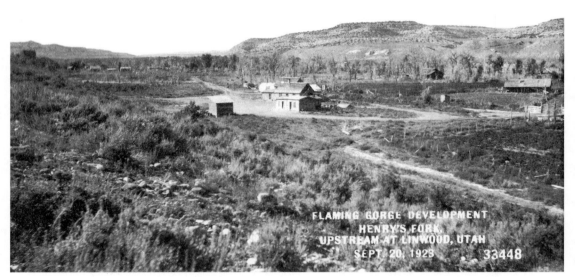

FLAMING GORGE DEVELOPMENT
HENRY'S FORK,
UPSTREAM AT LINWOOD, UTAH
SEPT. 20, 1923   33448

Linwood, Utah, 1923.

"The Fall of Cottonwoods"

The young man
Hesitates before stepping down
from his green government truck.
He needs to talk to Tom, to tell him
that tomorrow they will burn his barns and corrals;
bulldoze the barbed wire fences
and fell the cottonwoods that have aged
with him on the banks of Henry's Fork.
    "…the new dam is finished,
     and the lake is beginning to fill…"
Tom wears the rings of years in his face
and his gnarled hands have grown
stiff and brittle in the dry summer sun.
Wind-whipped and silent, he turns his back
to the young man and puppet-steps
down the long wooden porch and through
the warped door of his weathered home.
Inside the air smells strong of fruit
and must, undisturbed like the long neglected dust.

The young man promised to move the bunkhouse
and granary to higher ground,
but Bessie's grave and the copper mine
will never be found.
Finding the coffee pot cold, Tom shuffles
to the den where large, yellowed calendars
collage the gypsum walls. He pauses,
fingering a small one from the Linwood Merc.,
of the buildings burned the week before,
    "…the new dam is finished,
     and the lake is beginning to fill…"
Slumping into his cracked, leather chair
he lights his stubby cigar. The lingering smoke
curls into shape: A grey stallion—wild, free
and ready to run! Eyes closed, Tom fills his mind
with beating hooves…too full to hear
his son drive away
in the green government truck.

—Terry Lynn Jarvie Gardner

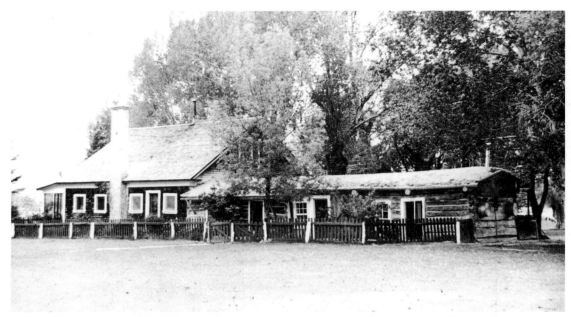

Keith Smith home, Linwood, Utah (Uncle Jack Robinson's cabin on far right). **Courtesy Barbara Williams Amburn.**

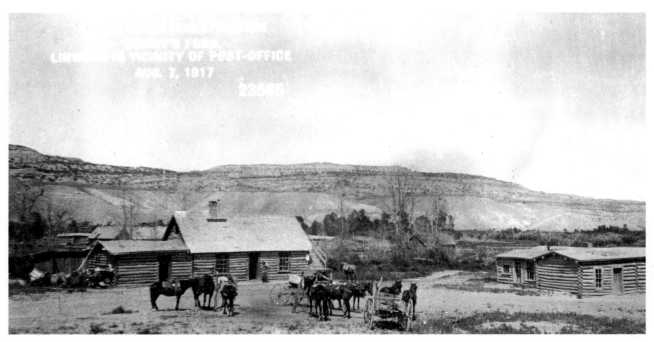

Linwood, Utah, 1917.

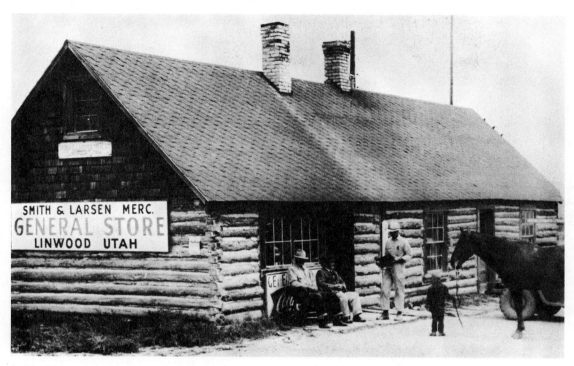

Smith and Larsen General Store, Linwood, Utah.

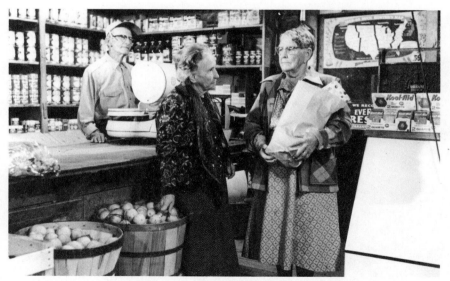

Inside Smith Larsen General Store (left to right: George Rasmussen, Minnie Crouse Rasmussen, unknown woman). *Courtesy Barbara Williams Amburn.*

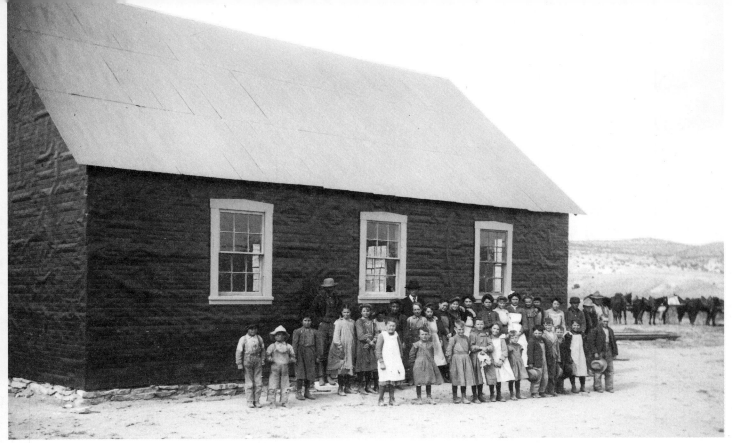

Linwood School, 1926. *Courtesy Sweetwater County Historical Museum.*

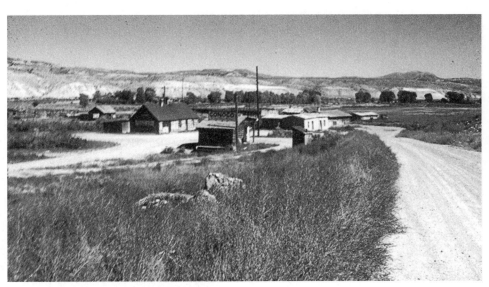

Linwood, Utah. *Courtesy Barbara Williams Amburn.*

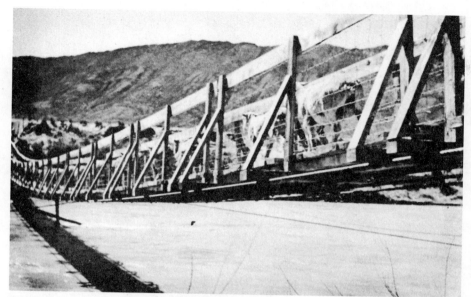

Keith Smith's suspension bridge, Linwood, Utah.

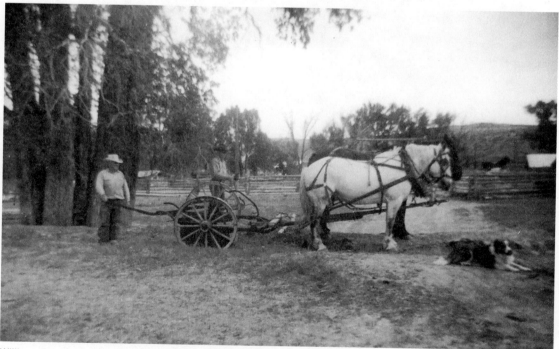

Williams Ranch, Henry's Fork. *Courtesy Barbara Williams Amburn.*

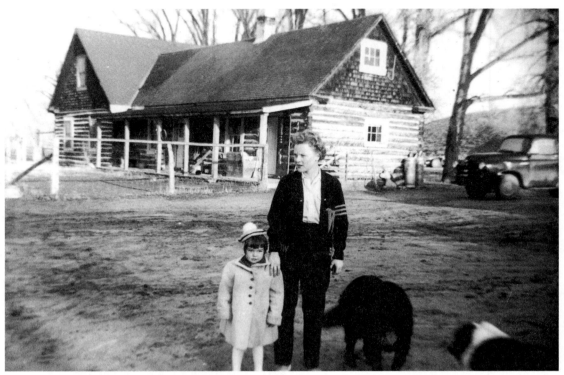

Williams Ranch, Henry's Fork. Courtesy Barbara Williams Amburn.

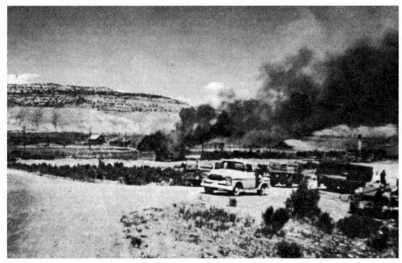

Linwood burning. *Courtesy Terry Lynn Jarvie Gardner.*

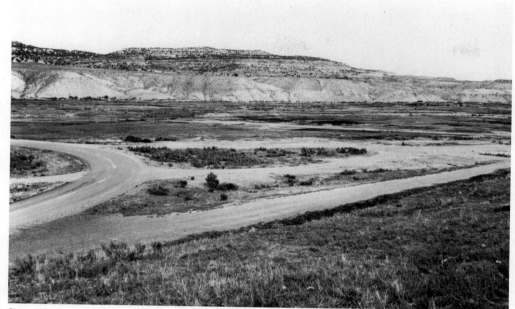

Site of Linwood after clearing. *Courtesy Barbara Williams Amburn.*

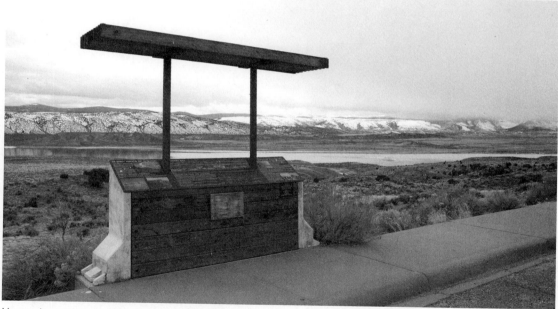

Linwood monument, with Linwood Bay in background.

NOTES

Chapter 1

1. James Clyman, *Journal of a Mountain Man*, August 29, 1844, 110. Like many of the early fur trade accounts, this has been reprinted fairly recently and is widely available.

2. Cutthroat trout (*Oncorhynchus clarkii*) is the only trout native to Utah. All others, including rainbow and brown trout, have been introduced. Steve Schmidt, owner of Western Rivers Flyfisher, telephone conversation, May 19, 2011.

3. These names, along with virtually all the names of significant features on the Green and Colorado Rivers from Green River, Wyoming, through the Grand Canyon, were bestowed by Major John Wesley Powell on his pioneering river voyages on the Green and Colorado in 1869 and 1871. A few local names, such as Nielson's Flat and Hideout Flat, survived, but most came from Powell's impressive vocabulary.

4. Geological information in this section comes from Douglas A. Sprinkel, *Geologic Guide along Flaming Gorge Reservoir, Flaming Gorge National Recreation Area, Utah–Wyoming.*

5. Today the Bureau of Reclamation rarely allows more than a fraction of that much water, usually about 1,000 to 3,000 cfs, to escape the dams. The next bridges downstream from the Green River railroad bridge would have been the Henry's Fork footbridge, built by Keith Smith and his family in the early 1900s, and the bridge built by the Civilian Conservation Corps (CCC) at Hideout Flat in the 1930s, both of which could carry sheep and cattle but not vehicles. The Swinging Bridge in Browns Park, which was the first place a car or truck could cross the river for over 120 miles downstream from Green River, was built in the 1920s. The frozen river was often used as a path for people and animals when deep snow closed the roads and trails.

6. William L. Purdy, oral interview, August 28, 1985.

7. Ellsworth Kolb, *Through the Grand Canyon from Wyoming to Mexico,* 29. Kolb may be taking some artistic license in placing roadrunners in the canyons of the upper Green. His book has been widely reprinted, in over forty editions. It's a delightful account of their pioneering voyage. In addition, the movie they made during the journey was shown at the Kolb studio on the South Rim of the Grand Canyon practically every day from their return until Emery's death in 1975, making it one of the longest-running motion pictures ever.

8. Dick Dunham to Otis Marston, September 16, 1977, Box 359, Folder 7, Otis Marston Papers, Huntington Library, San Marino, California.

9. Kent Day, *University of Utah Department of Anthropology Weekly Report,* July 15, 1962.

10. Fred Quartarone, *Historical Accounts of Upper Colorado River Basin Endangered Fish.* Ironically, before Flaming Gorge Dam was completed in 1963, these native fish were deemed "trash fish" and were all but wiped out by wildlife management agencies who were "paving the way for trout" in September 1962. See chapter 6.

11. Doyce B. Nunis, Jr., ed., *The Bidwell–Bartleson Party: 1841 California Emigrant Adventure,* 192.

12. Floyd Sharrock, *Prehistoric Occupation Patterns in Southwest Wyoming and Cultural Relationships with the Great Basin and Plains Culture Areas,* 148–50.

13. Steven R. Simms, *Ancient Peoples of the Great Basin and Colorado Plateau,* 141–67.

14. Kent C. Day and David S. Dibble, *Archaeological Survey of the Flaming Gorge Reservoir Area, Wyoming–Utah* (no. 65), 7.

15. Information on the Fremont comes from Richard K. Talbot and Lane D. Richens, *Fremont Farming and Mobility on the Far Northern Colorado Plateau;* Simms, *Ancient Peoples of the Great Basin and Colorado Plateau,* 185–222; and Richard K. Talbot and Lane D.

Richens, *Steinaker Gap: An Early Fremont Farmstead*, 177–80.

16. Rufus Wood Leigh, "Naming of the Green, Sevier, and Virgin Rivers," 137. I make this claim with no little trepidation, for the Shoshone origin of the name as "seedskeedee" has long been conventional wisdom in western historical circles. Yet the linguistic evidence as well as Leigh's article would seem to point toward a Crow origin. Unfortunately, Leigh does not cite his evidence for this assertion.

17. Warren L. D'Azevedo and William C. Sturtevant, eds., *Handbook of North American Indians*, vol. 11, *Great Basin*, 309.

18. Warren Angus Ferris, *Life in the Rocky Mountains*, 125. http://oghma.library.utah.edu:8991/F?func=item-global&doc_library=UUU01&local_base=UUU01&doc_number=000638580

19. Mae Urbanek, *Chief Washakie of the Shoshone*, 32.

20. Another name for the Green was the "Colorado River of the West." Even though no one really knew the course of the Green before 1869, people recognized that it had some connection with the Colorado River.

21. Hiram Chittenden, *The American Fur Trade of the Far West: A History of the Pioneer Trading Posts and Early Fur Companies of the Missouri Valley and the Rocky Mountains and of the Overland Commerce with Santa Fe*, 262. Chittenden's massive account (over a thousand pages) is one of the standard works on the history of the fur trade but hard to find outside libraries.

22. Dale Morgan, ed., *The West of William Ashley: The International Struggle for the Fur Trade of the Missouri, the Rocky Mountains, and the Columbia, with Explorations beyond the Continental Divide, Recorded in the Diaries and Letters of William H. Ashley and His Contemporaries, 1822–1838*, 106. Nathaniel Wyeth called it the "Sheckkskeedee," one of many variations of "Seeds-kee-dee."

23. Ibid. Thus did a simple business decision inaugurate the best-known institution of the fur trade, the rendezvous. This combination business convention, reunion, sporting competition, and bacchanal came to symbolize the era of the mountain men. Most of them were held somewhere near the Green River, until they died out with the collapse of the fur trade in the 1840s.

24. Harrison Clifford Dale, ed., *The Ashley-Smith Explorations and the Discovery of a Central Route to the Pacific, 1822–1829*, 140. Taken together, Morgan's and Dale's renditions of the Ashley journal and the Ashley narrative are the basis for documenting this important beginning of the fur trade on the Green River. Both are long out of print and only readily available in research libraries.

25. Dick Dunham and Vivian Dunham, *Flaming Gorge Country*, 98–100.

26. The cabin was located on land purchased by Keith Smith in what would become the town of Linwood; when Linwood was about to be covered by the waters of Flaming Gorge Reservoir, the cabin was dismantled and moved to Smith's new home near Greendale, Utah.

27. Nunis, *The Bidwell–Bartleson Party*, 244.

28. Ibid., 108–9.

29. Ibid., 83.

30. John Wesley Powell, *Exploration of the Colorado River and Its Canyons*, 131. Powell's expedition is not only one of the most written about explorations in the American West but also one of the best documented. Fortunately, the Utah State Historical Society and the University of Utah Press recently reissued the volumes of *Utah Historical Quarterly* that gather all the diaries, journals, and letters of the members of Powell's two expeditions in an easily available paperback set.

31. William Lewis Manly, *Death Valley in '49*, 1–53. One of the reasons Manly and his companions did not want to be left stranded in Salt Lake City was fear of the Mormons, who had recently been driven from Iowa, Illinois, and Missouri and were reputed to be very unfriendly toward anyone who came from those states. Manly, of course, was from New England; but the wagon train originated in Iowa, so guilt by association was enough to make him feel unwelcome. Manly's account is another early pioneer journal that has recently been reprinted and can be found in bookstores.

32. Ibid., 73–74.

33. Unlike Ashley's inscription, which became famous, no one ever reported seeing Manly's name in later years.

34. Manly, *Death Valley in '49*, 77–78.

35. Ibid.

36. Ibid. Manly's was not the only party of '49ers to try the river as an alternative. A few days later, in the Canyon of Lodore at a spot later identified by Powell as Disaster Falls, Manly found "a deserted camp, a skiff, and some heavy cooking utensils, with a notice posted on an alder tree saying that they had found the river route impracticable" (ibid., 79–80). Manly wrote down their names, but his journal was burned in a house fire some years later. By the time he wrote his memoir, he had forgotten them. No record exists of any other river travelers during the gold rush.

37. Robert Brewster Stanton, *Colorado River Controversies*, 174.

Chapter 2

1. Their caution was to little avail; the presence of Frenchmen—and especially an attractive young Frenchwoman—soon became front-page news in all the newspapers along the river and in other regional papers as well. The French kayakers were in the news in those days, but their story is little known outside Colorado River history circles. One source is Roy Webb, "Les Voyageurs Sans Trace: The DeColmont-DeSeyne Kayak Party of 1938."

2. Those license plates are still on Nevills's boat, which is now part of the Historic Boats collection of Grand Canyon National Park. Expedition Island NHS is still maintained by the city of Green River as a park and picnic area. The island has three stone monuments to Powell. In the 1990s I was asked to write text for a number of monuments to be placed on a walking path around the little island that would commemorate other river voyagers. The dedication of those informational signs was also the occasion for a city-wide celebration.

3. William Purdy, *An Outline of the History of the Flaming Gorge Area*, 15. Purdy, a native of the coal town of Superior, Wyoming, grew up with a view of the Green River basin. As a student at the University of Utah he wanted to write a master's thesis on the history of the Uinta Mountains and the Green River. He was advised to move to the area to immerse himself in the history and took the job as principal of the school in Manila, Utah. While living there he became fascinated with the history of the area and the Green River. Though he never wrote the master's thesis, he

did become immersed in local history and lore. He purchased a folding kayak so that he could float down the Green and probably spent more time in those canyons than any other person before or since. Later he moved to Salt Lake City to teach at St. Mark's Prep School for Boys, where he spent the rest of his teaching career.

4. Roy Webb, ed., *High, Wide, and Handsome: The River Journals of Norman D. Nevills*, 189. Nevills was an inveterate journal keeper and typed up his notes made during summer river trips in much expanded form during the long winters in his home in Mexican Hat, Utah. This volume gathers all those journals of his major trips in one book and annotates them through use of his extensive correspondence, housed in Manuscripts Collection MS552 in the Special Collections Department, J. Willard Marriott Library, University of Utah.

5. Ellsworth Kolb, *Through the Grand Canyon from Wyoming to Mexico*, 13. In 1922 the Logan Ranch was known as the Teter Ranch.

6. Doris Nevills, "Woman Conquerors of the Colorado."

7. Webb, *High, Wide, and Handsome*, 64.

8. Galloway-Stone Expedition, Collected Journals. This compilation of accounts by all members of the 1909 expedition does not differentiate who wrote this particular passage. The only published account by a member of this party was Julius F. Stone's *Canyon Country: The Romance of a Drop of Water and a Grain of Sand*. A copy of Galloway's journal was deposited in the Special Collections Department, J. Willard Marriott Library, University of Utah, and is available online, along with 100 photographs by Raymond Cogswell. Both were donated by descendants of the members of the party.

9. Douglas A. Sprinkel, *Geologic Guide along Flaming Gorge Reservoir, Flaming Gorge National Recreation Area, Utah-Wyoming*, 7. The Green River Formation is also famous for fish and plant fossils, such as those found at Fossil Butte National Monument.

10. Cid Ricketts Sumner, *Traveler in the Wilderness*, 45–46. Cid Sumner, author of the "Tammy" series of books for young girls, was seventy years old when she signed up for the Eggert-Hatch Film Expedition in 1955.

11. Box 288, Folder 1, Otis Marston Papers, Huntington Library, San Marino, California. An article in the *Green River Star* described them as "one day sashays through Firehole."
12. Lee Roy Brinegar, telephone conversation, December 3, 2010.
13. Kolb, *Through the Grand Canyon from Wyoming to Mexico*, 16–17.
14. Antoine de Seynes, 1938, ACCN 1206. In the films taken by the French kayakers (A0531) now in the Multimedia Archives, Special Collections, University of Utah, Geneviève is shown riding a horse on the Holmes Ranch, wearing a ten-gallon hat. One of the few to decline the Holmes Ranch hospitality was the USGS/Utah Power and Light survey party in 1922. Ralf Woolley, the leader, felt that his large crew of surveyors and boatmen would be an "imposition."
15. Obituary for Emma Holmes, *Green River Star*, July 17, 1958. She lived at the ranch until 1954, when her health necessitated a move to Green River.
16. Webb, *High, Wide, and Handsome*, 65.
17. Ibid., 190.
18. Maradel Marston, Journal. Otis Marston was known as "Dock." Maradel was his daughter; her twin, Loel, was also along on the trip.
19. Otis Marston to Phil Lundstrom, February 16, 1952, Box 120, Folder 23, Otis Marston Papers, Huntington Library, San Marino, California.
20. *Green River Star*, June 6, 1952, 8.
21. Purdy, *An Outline of the History of the Flaming Gorge Area*, 29–30. Also http://www.wyomingtalesandtrails.com/griver2.html (October 13, 2008).
22. Dick Dunham and Vivian Dunham, *Flaming Gorge Country*, 311; interview with Barbara Williams Amburn, March 16, 2011.
23. Ralf R. Woolley, "A Boat Trip Down Green River from Green River, Wyo.–Green River, Ut., July 10–Sept 14 1922," 8.
24. Lee Roy Brinegar, telephone conversation, December 3, 2010. When William Brinegar died around 1950, his son Lee Roy took over the ranch. He ran it until forced to sell by the Bureau of Reclamation in 1963.
25. Warren Angus Ferris, *Life in the Rocky Mountains*, 38.
26. Woolley, "A Boat Trip Down Green River from Green River, Wyo.–Green River, Ut.," 9.
27. Mary Beckwith, Journal (1956).
28. Woolley, "A Boat Trip Down Green River from Green River, Wyo.–Green River, Ut.," #21, 8.
29. Ralf Woolley, *The Green River and Its Utilization*, 40. Besides the technical data gathered by Woolley, this hard-to-find document contains a summation of the known exploration of the Green River up to the time of publication as well as a detailed narrative of the 1922 survey.
30. John Wesley Powell, *Exploration of the Colorado River and Its Canyons*, 11.
31. Michael W. Johnson, *A History of Daggett County: A Modern Frontier*, 84–85. Johnson's book, one of the Utah Statehood Centennial Series, contains a wealth of information about the area along the Green River from the Utah state boundary to Browns Park. The chapter on the Flaming Gorge Dam is especially good, but the entire book is well worth reading.
32. Dunham and Dunham, *Flaming Gorge Country*, 141–44.
33. Interview with Barbara Williams Amburn, March 16, 2011; and telephone conversation, June 1, 2011.
34. Two good and easily accessible sources on Linwood's colorful history are Johnson's *History of Daggett County*, which also covers the Lucerne Land and Water Company and other irrigation efforts; and Doris Karren Burton's *Settlements of Uintah County: Digging Deeper*. Dunham and Dunham's *Flaming Gorge Country* is engaging but sadly unsourced. Keith Smith's "Recollections of Keith Smith of Linwood, Utah, as Told to His Daughter Susan" is detailed and personal but only available in archives. Carma Potter McDowell's *Linwood Resurrected: A Town Buried under the Flaming Gorge Lake* was likewise privately published and is not easily available. The history of Linwood was widely covered in local newspapers, however, when it was being torn down.
35. Smith, "Recollections of Keith Smith of Linwood, Utah, as Told to His Daughter Susan," 10.
36. The bridge over Henry's Fork lasted until 1955, when it was replaced by a steel bridge. McDowell, *Linwood Resurrected*, 9.
37. Smith, "Recollections of Keith Smith of Linwood, Utah, as Told to His Daughter Susan," 8–11.
38. Linwood was a local name for cottonwood trees, rows of which had been planted by George Solomon. John W. Van Cott, *Utah Place Names: A Comprehensive*

Guide to the Origins of Geographic Names—A Compilation, 227–28.

39. "70 Year Old Linwood Post Office Ends," *Green River Star,* October 1962, Special Collections, J. Willard Marriott Library, University of Utah.

40. Dunham and Dunham, *Flaming Gorge Country,* 138–43. Sheep were kept out of the Henry's Fork country by cattle ranchers, who established a "dead line" north of there. Sheep that crossed over that line were killed. This practice faded away by the turn of the twentieth century.

41. http://www.wyomingtalesandtrails.com/photos4a.html (October 13, 2008).

42. Dunham and Dunham, *Flaming Gorge Country,* 138–43.

43. Roy Webb, *If We Had A Boat: Green River Explorers, Adventurers, and Runners,* 104. Also http://www.wyomingtalesandtrails.com/griver2.html (October 2, 2009).

44. Interview with Barbara Williams Amburn, March 16, 2011.

Chapter 3

1. Douglas A. Sprinkel, *Geologic Guide along Flaming Gorge Reservoir, Flaming Gorge National Recreation Area, Utah–Wyoming,* 12–16.

2. F. E. Shearer, ed., *The Pacific Tourist: Adams & Bishop's Illustrated Trans-continental Guide of Travel, from the Atlantic to the Pacific Ocean,* 101.

3. Ralf Woolley, *The Green River and Its Utilization,* 40–41.

4. Frederick S. Dellenbaugh, *A Canyon Voyage: The Narrative of the Second Powell Expedition Down the Green & Colorado Rivers,* 17.

5. Interview with Barbara Williams Amburn, March 16, 2011.

6. This would have given this section of river a fall of around 40 feet per mile, far more than the actual drop in Red Canyon, which is about 13 feet per mile. The greatest fall of any of the canyons of the Green River is 21.7 feet per mile, downstream in Split Mountain Canyon.

7. James P. Beckwourth, *The Life and Adventures of James P. Beckwourth,* 59–60.

8. Ellsworth Kolb, *Through the Grand Canyon from Wyoming to Mexico,* 20. In 1989, as I was preparing for a lengthy river trip in Green River, Wyoming, that would commemorate John Wesley Powell's voyage, a major storm caused big waves on Flaming Gorge Reservoir that swamped several power boats. Consequently, we were told by a number of local residents that Flaming Gorge Reservoir and the river below were too dangerous to navigate and that we would surely come to grief, even though people had been doing it for well over 150 years. It was the latter-day version of the "Green River Suck."

9. Haldane "Buzz" Holmstrom, Diary (1937). An excellent published biography of Buzz Holmstrom is Brad Dimock, Vince Welch, and Cort Conley, *The Doing of the Thing: The Brief, Brilliant Whitewater Career of Buzz Holmstrom.*

10. John Wesley Powell, *Exploration of the Colorado River and Its Canyons,* 14.

11. Otis R. "Dock" Marston, "Notes on Green River Trip, 1947."

12. Roy Webb, ed., *High, Wide, and Handsome: The River Journals of Norman D. Nevills,* 191.

13. Mary Beckwith, Journal (1956). Frederick S. Dellenbaugh, who accompanied Powell on his 1871 voyage and later became his hagiographer, was typically defensive about Powell's overblown description. In a letter to Julius Stone, he wrote: "I don't think Powell meant to refer 'conspicuously' to the little rapid in Horseshoe Canyon. We all noted it, not because it amounted to anything as a rapid, but simply because it was the place where the river changed its mood. Thenceforward the character was different." Dellenbaugh to Julius Stone, March 24, 1932, Box 359, Folder 19, Otis Marston Papers, Huntington Library, San Marino, California.

14. Keith Smith, "Recollections of Keith Smith of Linwood, Utah, as Told to His Daughter Susan," 10–11.

15. Doris Karren Burton, *Settlements of Uintah County: Digging Deeper,* 534.

16. Ralf R. Woolley, "A Boat Trip Down Green River from Green River, Wyo.–Green River, Ut., July 10–Sept 14 1922," 8, 10–11. When the dam was being built, this house and all of its improvements would have been razed or burned.

17. Webb, *High, Wide, and Handsome,* 66.

18. *A Field Guide to Birds of North America* (New York: Golden Press, 1966), 178.

19. Powell, *Exploration of the Colorado River and Its Canyons*, 15. Of these charming names, only Kingfisher Canyon has lasted. Kingfisher Creek is now known as Sheep Creek, while the little park at the mouth of Sheep Creek is now under Flaming Gorge Reservoir.

20. Marston's notes on interview with Frank Swain, May 29, 1948, Box 225, Folder 1, Otis Marston Papers, Huntington Library, San Marino, California.

21. Roy Webb, *Riverman: The Story of Bus Hatch*, 25.

22. One such flood on the night of June 9–10, 1965, killed a family of seven people who were camping in Sheep Creek Canyon. This same storm caused a major debris flow on the Yampa River that enlarged Warm Springs rapid; the first boatman who tried to run it was thrown from his boat and drowned.

23. Amos Burg, Postcards, September 6, 1938.

24. Powell, *Exploration of the Colorado River and Its Canyons*, 15.

25. Ellsworth Kolb, *Through the Grand Canyon from Wyoming to Mexico*, 41–44. Hideout Flat is one of the few local names not bestowed by John Wesley Powell.

26. Oral interview with A. K. Reynolds, October 12, 2003. Members of the CCC also built the Sheep Creek footbridge as well as a trail down the river on the right side that went to Eagle Creek and followed it to Green Lakes Lodge, which is still in business, now known as Red Canyon Lodge.

27. Dellenbaugh, *A Canyon Voyage*, 22.

28. Woolley, *The Green River and Its Utilization*, 56. Only Split Mountain Canyon has a greater fall per mile.

29. *Grand Valley Times*, December 4, 1896.

30. Charles Kelly, ed., "Captain Francis Marion Bishop's Journal: August 15, 1870–June 3, 1872," 169.

31. Ibid. Richardson decided that he had experienced enough adventure and left the party at Browns Park. The incident is covered in all of the Powell party journals from 1871 as well as in Dellenbaugh's later books.

32. Marjorie Steurt, [no title], *Southland Federal Savings Magazine* 5, no. 2 (April 1957), Box 206, Folder 4, Otis Marston Papers, Huntington Library, San Marino California.

33. "List of River Touring Section Trips, 1960," *Sierra Club Bulletin* (February 1960): 10.

34. Woolley, "A Boat Trip Down Green River from Green River, Wyo.–Green River, Ut.," 13.

35. Cid Ricketts Sumner, *Traveler in the Wilderness*, 62–63.

36. Albert "Bert" Loper to H. E. Blake, July 7, 1940.

37. Ken Sleight, oral interview, October 21, 2003. In those days many river runners hunted for geese and deer.

38. *St. Louis Republic*, June 1909.

39. Box 278, Folder 4, Otis Marston Papers, Huntington Library, San Marino, California, contains a number of articles written both before and after their abortive journey as well as other information about their ill-fated trip. One source says that they were lost for four days before they met the Indian and were naked when they were discovered cowering in Keith Smith's blacksmith shop in Linwood.

40. Kolb, *Through the Grand Canyon from Wyoming to Mexico*, 5–6.

41. Woolley, "A Boat Trip Down Green River from Green River, Wyo.–Green River, Ut.," 14.

42. Helen Kendall, Journal (1960).

43. William L. Tennent, *John Jarvie of Browns Park*.

44. Dellenbaugh, *A Canyon Voyage*, 25. It is hard not to detect a note of self-satisfaction in Dellenbaugh's writing about Hook's unfortunate demise.

45. Buried next to Hook at the Jarvie Ranch is Jesse Ewing, who was apparently with Hook on the fateful voyage but survived to start mining in Browns Park and develop a very unsavory reputation for draining his partners of money and then finding an excuse to murder them. He was later killed in an altercation over a Madame Forrestal, a former contortionist.

46. Albert "Bert" Loper, "Notes of Bert Loper for 1922."

47. I have yet to find a reference to why Gold Point is so named. A gold claim was apparently filed there at one point for a placer deposit, and a table in the *Salt Lake Mining Review* noted $20,000 worth of ore taken out of "Red Canyon," but solid information about it is so far lacking.

48. Woolley, "A Boat Trip Down Green River from Green River, Wyo.–Green River, Ut.," 17–18.

49. http://www.prospector-utah.com/brown.htm (January 12, 2011). This website is unfortunately devoid of any bibliography or notes on sources. The author claims that Hill moved to Vernal when he got too old and died there. Hill is listed in the Utah Cemetery and Burial database as having been born

in 1851 and is buried in the Rock Point Cemetery near Vernal.

50. William L. Purdy, oral interview, August 28, 1985.

Chapter 4

1. William Lewis Manly, *Death Valley in '49*, 75.
2. Ibid., 79–80. Manly had just painted his own name with a mixture of gunpowder and tar on a cliff upstream from Ashley Falls.
3. Manly's *Death Valley in '49* was first published in 1896; Harrison Clifford Dale, ed., *The Ashley-Smith Explorations and the Discovery of a Central Route to the Pacific, 1822–1829* in 1918.
4. Frederick S. Dellenbaugh, *The Romance of the Colorado River*, 110–11. Dellenbaugh was only seventeen when he went on the epic journey with Powell in 1871 as the trip's artist and can thus be forgiven if he devoted himself to hero worship of the major for the rest of his life. Dellenbaugh became Powell's chronicler, defender, and apologist—hagiographer would not be too strong a word. His wrote widely on a number of western topics, but his two books on Powell and his explorations are *The Romance of the Colorado River* and *A Canyon Voyage*. Both are still available in modern editions. They are detailed and well-written accounts worth reading for an insider's view of Powell, albeit through rose-colored glasses. *A Canyon Voyage* was also the first book to bring to light Powell's 1871 trip and its crew, which Powell had famously ignored when he wrote his report in 1871. Dellenbaugh maintained a long and fruitful correspondence with many figures in Colorado River history until his death in 1935.
5. John Wesley Powell, *Exploration of the Colorado River and Its Canyons*, 142–43. Ashley remained an enigma until well into the twentieth century.
6. [Russell Frazier, no title], *Outdoor Life* (September 1937): 21.
7. Ellsworth Kolb, *Through the Grand Canyon from Wyoming to Mexico*, 38–39.
8. Almon Harris Thompson, "Diary of Almon Harris Thompson," 16.
9. George Y. Bradley, "George Y. Bradley's Journal," 33.
10. Stephen Vandiver Jones, "Journal of Stephen Vandiver Jones," 32.
11. Ibid.

12. John F. Steward, "Journal of John F. Steward," 188.
13. Frederick S. Dellenbaugh, *A Canyon Voyage: The Narrative of the Second Powell Expedition Down the Green & Colorado Rivers*, 27.
14. Ibid., 28.
15. Roy Webb, *If We Had A Boat: Green River Explorers, Adventurers, and Runners*, 87–89.
16. George F. Flavell, *The Log of the Panthon*, 19. Galloway was on the river at the same time as Flavell, and the two men met up in Needles, California, in the winter of 1897. When Flavell asked Galloway what he thought of the trip, he replied that it was "of little profit." Flavell's *Log* is getting harder to find but is a required addition to any river library for its self-effacing charm and energy.
17. Nathaniel Galloway, Papers, diary entry for September 18, 1909.
18. Kolb, *Through the Grand Canyon from Wyoming to Mexico*, 37–38.
19. Ralf R. Woolley, "A Boat Trip Down Green River from Green River, Wyo.–Green River, Ut., July 10–Sept 14 1922," 18–19. The photographs are found in P0563 in the Marriott Library Special Collections Department. The 1922 survey trip is also recounted in Pearl Baker, *Trail on the Water*, a biography of Bert Loper; and Dick Westwood, *Rough-Water Man: Elwyn Blake's Colorado River Expeditions*.
20. Blake was a second-generation riverman. His father, H. E. Blake, Sr., had been a pioneer steamboater on the Green and Colorado between Green River and Moab, Utah, around the turn of the twentieth century.
21. F. LeMoyne Page, "My Trip Down the Green River," 5. Page, however, says that they ran the rapid only after "considerable study." Sources for this trip include H. Elwyn Blake, "Diary of H. Elwyn Blake Jr."; and Westwood, *Rough-Water Man*.
22. Quotations from Holmstrom's diaries courtesy of Brad Dimock, co-author of *The Doing of the Thing: The Brief, Brilliant Whitewater Career of Buzz Holmstrom*.
23. See note 22 above. Burg's boat, the *Charlie*, was specially made to his design by the Goodrich Rubber Company and was the first inflatable boat specifically designed for running rapids. It also became the first inflatable boat to run Ashley Falls.

24. "A Journal of Antoine de Seynes," entry for September 20, 1938, translated from French original by Terry Fahey.

25. Stewart Gardiner interview by Roy Webb, July 17, 1984, ACCN 1000, Special Collections Department, J. Willard Marriott Library, University of Utah.

26. Roy Webb, ed., *High, Wide, and Handsome: The River Journals of Norman D. Nevills*, 67.

27. Ibid., 192–93. Nevills was also suffering from severe food poisoning that he had gotten the day before. His 1949 journal was lost after his death in an airplane crash on September 19, 1949.

28. Harry Aleson, "Notes on Green River Trip, 1951," 5. Several photos of some of the inscriptions are found in the Otis Marston Papers at the Huntington Library in San Marino, California.

29. Frederick Dellenbaugh to Julius F. Stone, May 29, 1929, Box 359, Folder 28, Otis Marston Papers, Huntington Library, San Marino, California.

30. William L. Purdy, oral interview, August 28, 1985.

31. Laphene "Don" Harris, oral interview, March 14, 1990.

32. *Water Resources Bulletin* (Feb. 1947): 59–61. In his oral interview in October 2004, A. K. Reynolds recounted another story about one of his friends capsizing in Ashley Falls, but he quickly recovered in the big pool below the rapid. His wife, Ellen Reynolds, says that she was the one who fell out of the boat and had to be picked up below.

33. Cal Giddings, oral interview, July 3, 1984.

Chapter 5

1. John W. Van Cott, *Utah Place Names: A Comprehensive Guide to the Origins of Geographic Names—A Compilation*, 119. Also http://www.daggettcounty.org/index.aspx?nid=57 (January 16, 2011). Van Cott says that Honselena was from Prussia.

2. Dick DeJournette and Daun DeJournette, *One Hundred Years of Browns Park and Diamond Mountain*, 269–70. Kerry Ross Boren spins a great number of tales about Dutch John's outlaw exploits at this interesting but unfortunately unsourced website: http://www.prospector-utah.com/brown.htm (January 16, 2011).

3. Jack Hillers, *"Photographed All the Best Scenery": Jack Hiller's Diary of the Powell Expeditions, 1871–1875*, 30. Hillers was originally hired as a teamster but later taught himself how to operate a glass plate camera and became the expedition's official photographer.

4. "William C. Richmond's Story of His Trip through the Grand Canyon with Nathaniel Galloway in 1897," Box 198, Folder 6, Otis Marston Papers, Huntington Library, San Marino, California. Richmond left a very entertaining account of the voyage in this document.

5. J. Neil Murdock, *Early History of the Colorado River Storage Project*, 1. Little Hole is also where the opening scenes of the movie *Jeremiah Johnson*, starring Robert Redford, were filmed in 1972. Today it's a popular campground for hikers, boaters, and fishers along the heavily used stretch of the Green below Flaming Gorge Dam.

6. DeJournette and DeJournette, *One Hundred Years of Browns Park and Diamond Mountain*, 239–43. During his final illness, Williams moved to Vernal, Utah, and lived with Frank Hatch, father of famous riverman Bus Hatch. Despite the disapproval of his neighbors, who did not want a black man in their neighborhood, Frank nursed Williams until he died in May 1934 and saw to his burial in Vernal's Rock Point Cemetery.

7. Doris Karren Burton, *Behind Swinging Doors: Colorful History of Uinta Basin*, 187. One of Orsen Burton's sons, Jesse "Shorty" Burton, worked as a river guide for Hatch River Expeditions and was famous for the quality of his dutch-oven cooking, which he learned in his father's sheep camps. He drowned when his boat overturned in the Grand Canyon in 1967. Burton's books, including *Settlements of Uintah County: Digging Deeper* and *Behind Swinging Doors*, are outgrowths of her entry in the Utah Statehood Centennial County History Series, *A History of Uintah County: Scratching the Surface*.

8. Marjorie Steurt, "Diary of Green River Trip—1955 September." Little Hole was finally acquired by the Utah Division of Wildlife Resources in 1978.

9. DeJournette and DeJournette, *One Hundred Years of Browns Park and Diamond Mountain*, 265–67.

10. Thomas Jefferson Farnham, *Travels in the Great Western Prairies*, 62.

11. C. C. Sharp, "Notes on Colorado River Trip."

12. Nathaniel Galloway, "Diary of the Galloway-Stone Expedition," 6.

13. Albert "Bert" Loper, "Notes of Bert Loper for 1922." Loper, the "Grand Old Man of the Colorado,"

features largely in early accounts of river travel on the Colorado River system. A recent biography of him is available: Brad Dimock, *The Very Hard Way: Bert Loper and the Colorado River*.

14. F. Lemoyne Page, "My Trip Down the Green River," 6.

15. H. Elwyn Blake, "Boating the Wild Rivers," 155. Later, after all the big rapids had been run, "Og" West managed to pin one of the boats irretrievably on a rock in mid-channel in the Canyon of Lodore; they were forced to abandon it. Parley Galloway, Nathaniel's ne'er-do-well son, later retrieved it and sold it to Hod Ruple in Island Park, where it was seen by Bus Hatch. The well-built boat became the model for a subsequent fleet of boats built by Bus and his friends and used extensively to run rivers until after World War II.

16. Brad Dimock, ed., *Every Rapid Speaks Plainly: The Salmon, Green, and Colorado River Journals of Buzz Holmstrom*, 39–40. Holmstrom portaged only three more times, twice in Lodore and once in Cataract Canyon. The next year, when he ran the same trip with Amos Burg, he ran every rapid all the way through the Grand Canyon, the first person ever to do so.

17. At the same time Norman Nevills was taking his first commercial passengers down the river on the lower Green, on the way to Cataract Canyon and ultimately the Grand Canyon.

18. Antoine de Seynes, Papers.

19. Ibid., #17.

20. Helen Kendall, Journal.

21. All books about Browns Park mention John Jarvie, but the best treatment of the man himself is William L. Tennent's *John Jarvie of Browns Park*. Browns Park today is much more sparsely populated than it was a hundred years ago, but the public's interest in this remote valley itself seems inexhaustible. The mystery of the outlaws, the drama of the struggles between ranchers and sheep herders, and the tales of the trappers in the park are part of the warp and woof of the American West. The result has been an outpouring of books, articles, websites, and documentaries. Some writing is better than the rest, but all of it is entertaining and interesting for those so inclined. Several of the better books are listed in the bibliography.

22. Michael W. Johnson, *A History of Daggett County: A Modern Frontier*, 254–55.

Chapter 6

1. Bureau of Reclamation, *The Colorado River: A Natural Menace Becomes a National Resource* (Washington, D.C.: Government Printing Office, 1946).

2. Michael W. Johnson, *A History of Daggett County: A Modern Frontier*, 190.

3. Marston MSS, Box 280, Folder 22, Otis Marston Papers, Huntington Library, San Marino, California.

4. The Colorado River Compact was finally signed at Santa Fe in October 1922 after years of tense negotiations, akin to a treaty between warring states. Secretary of commerce and future president Herbert Hoover was the chief negotiator. Serious flaws in the provisions came to light almost immediately: the quantity of water was much less than supposed, and what about Mexico? Some states did not sign the compact until the 1940s. It remains a source of much contention among the Colorado River basin states to this day. This incredibly complex topic has kept legions of attorneys employed for decades and can be hard to dig into. John Upton Terrell, *War for the Colorado River*, despite its dramatic title, is the most detailed academic version of this story. Marc Reisner's *Cadillac Desert* also covers it well in telling the whole story of the development of the Colorado River.

5. Ralf Woolley, *The Green River and Its Utilization*, 40. I go into some detail on the 1922 Green River survey in my book *If We Had A Boat: Green River Explorers, Adventurers, and Runners*. The story of the river surveys is also told in Dick Westwood's enjoyable book about his uncle: *Rough-Water Man: Elwyn Blake's Colorado River Expeditions*. Blake, whose father H. E. Blake, Sr., had been a pioneer steamboater on the lower Green, was a boatman on the Green, San Juan, and Grand Canyon surveys. Bert Loper's role in the 1921 San Juan and 1922 Green River surveys is covered in detail in Brad Dimock, *The Very Hard Way: Bert Loper and the Colorado River*. For a full history of the USGS surveys of the 1920s, see Bob Webb and Diane Boyer, *Damming Grand Canyon: The 1923 USGS Colorado River Expedition*, which concentrates on the Grand Canyon but gives a good overview of all the surveys.

6. The photographs of the 1922 survey are included in the more than 15,000 photographs donated by Utah Power and Light to the Special Collections Department, J. Willard Marriott Library, University of Utah, in the early 1970s. The originals were nitrate negatives, which are dangerously unstable, so a private donor financed the printing of each one. They are housed as collection P0206 and are available for the public to view.

7. Only two others, Split Mountain Dam and Rattlesnake Dam in Gray Canyon, were ever seriously considered. The Split Mountain Dam was quietly dropped when the Echo Park Dam was deleted from the Colorado River Storage Project. The Rattlesnake Dam, in soft, fractured rock above Green River, Utah, was an obvious disaster waiting to happen, so it too was shelved.

8. The Echo Park Dam controversy, as the first major defeat of the dam builders by a grassroots citizens' campaign, has received a great deal of attention from historians and scholars. One of the best books about it is Mark Harvey's *A Symbol of Wilderness: Echo Park and the American Conservation Movement*. Another is Jon M. Cosco, *Echo Park: Struggle for Preservation*. Wallace Earle Stegner, ed., *This Is Dinosaur: Echo Park Country and Its Magic Rivers* is a contemporary coffee table book of stunning photographs that helped turn public opinion against the dam.

9. Don Harris had only had small wooden skiffs called cataract boats; by this time Bus Hatch, who had outfitted numerous anti- and pro-dam groups down the Green during the Echo Park Dam controversy, had big surplus pontoons that could haul large parties, heavy equipment such as drilling rigs, and supplies.

10. J. Neil Murdock, *Early History of the Colorado River Storage Project*, 1. This book is a little hard to find, but it's a comprehensive, detailed history of the building of the dam. Murdock was an engineer for the Bureau of Reclamation.

11. A similar flood came down the Colorado, resulting in one of the largest floods in recorded history going through the Grand Canyon. The combined rivers rose to over 125,000 cfs.

12. Personal communication (name unknown), March 11, 2011.

13. Ted Hatch, oral history interview, August 7, 2003.

14. Mary Beckwith, Journal (1956).

15. L. C. B. McCullough, Journal, May 13, 1959.

16. *Desert Magazine* (June 1959): 20.

17. Wonderland Expeditions brochure (1962), Box 210, Folder 1, Otis Marston Papers, Huntington Library, San Marino, California. Sleight, an engaging and committed if sometimes quixotic environmentalist, was also one of the few people to oppose the Glen Canyon Dam while it was being built and served as the model for the character of Seldom Seen Smith in Edward Abbey's classic *cri de coeur The Monkey Wrench Gang*.

18. Ted Hatch, oral history interview, August 7, 2003.

19. Four of these documents were published in the University of Utah Anthropological Papers series. The two biological surveys are Seville Flowers, *Ecological Studies of the Flora and Fauna of Flaming Gorge Reservoir Basin, Utah and Wyoming* (no. 48); and Seville Flowers, *Vegetation of Flaming Gorge Reservoir Basin* (no. 43).

20. Dee Ann Story (1931–2010), http://www.legacy. com/obituaries/statesman/obituary.aspx?n=dee-ann-story&pid=147473057 (June 4, 2011).

21. Dr. Jesse Jennings to William Purdy, June 19, 1958, Department of Anthropology Records, 1937–97, ACCN 499, University of Utah Archives and Records Management.

22. Dr. Jesse Jennings to William Purdy, July 21, 1958.

23. William Purdy to Dr. Jesse Jennings, July 28, 1958.

24. Dr. Jesse Jennings to William Purdy, August 5, 1958.

25. Charlie R. Steen to Dr. Jesse Jennings, April 15, 1959.

26. Kent Day, *University of Utah Department of Anthropology Weekly Report*, July 28, 1962.

27. Dr. Jesse Jennings, "Attachment to the Flaming Gorge Report," January 22, 1959.

28. William Purdy, *An Outline of the History of the Flaming Gorge Area* (no. 37). The many other photos and some collections of artifacts and charcoal currently languish in the Department of Anthropology at the University of Utah.

29. Dick Dunham and Vivian Dunham, *Flaming Gorge Country*, 335–36, quoted in Michael W. Johnson, *A History of Daggett County: A Modern Frontier*, 216.

30. Interview with Barbara Williams Amburn, March 16, 2011.

31. According to Alonzo Jarvie, Lee Roy Brinegar was "the hardest to work with; he wouldn't even talk to us." See note 33 below.

32. Virtually all of the buildings that were saved from ranches or from Linwood are on private land, and permission is required to see any of them. Travelers should inquire locally in Manila, Dutch John, or the Flaming Gorge Resort about the possibility of seeing the Linwood school or other buildings before attempting to visit them.

33. The story of the last days of Linwood is also told in Carol Lynn Terry (Alonzo Jarvie's daughter), "The Day Linwood Burned," *Empire: Magazine of the Denver Post*, October 15, 1978, 42–45. Minnie Crouse Rasmussen did return eventually; after her death in Arizona, she was buried in the tiny cemetery at Minnie's Gap, east of Flaming Gorge Reservoir. Alonzo Jarvie was haunted by memories of the process of moving people away from their homes, including his own father, Tom Jarvie.

34. "List of River Touring Section Trips," *Sierra Club Bulletin* (February 1960): 10.

35. Don Hatch, oral interview, March 10, 1984.

36. "Echo Park Dam Will Create a Playground for Millions!" (n.d.) (copy in author's possession).

37. "Senator Frank Moss Seeks Bill for 'Lake Kennedy,'" *Vernal Express*, December 5, 1963.

38. Letter to the editor by Ken Sleight of Wonderland Expeditions, *Salt Lake Tribune*, January 19, 1963.

39. Ken Sleight to Otis Marston, February 4, 1963, Box 210, Folder 1, Otis Marston Papers, Huntington Library, San Marino California.

40. "Retain Memory of Linwood" [unknown newspaper, no date], Special Collections, J. Willard Marriott Library, University of Utah.

41. [unknown newspaper, no date], Box 359, Folder 33, Otis Marston Papers, Huntington Library, San Marino, California.

42. Fred Quartarone, *Historical Accounts of Upper Colorado River Basin Endangered Fish*, 37–48. Johnson's *History of Daggett County* also contains information on the fish kill (217–18). Another factor in their decline was the introduction of catfish into the Green in the 1930s. The river is perfect habitat for the catfish, which flourished. The larger pikeminnow would swallow a catfish, which would then extend its dorsal spines, lodging the smaller fish in its throat and causing both to die slowly. Ironically, these very same fish are now the focus of a great deal of effort to save them from extinction. Today these fish survive only in relict populations in the Yampa River, in the Green below the Uinta Basin, and at the mouth of the Little Colorado River in the Grand Canyon.

43. Johnson, *A History of Daggett County*, 218.

44. "Flaming Gorge Recreation Area Bill Signed by President," *Vernal Express*, October 3, 1968.

45. "Pipeline Controversy: Tapping the Green River," *Salt Lake Tribune* (online edition: http://www.sltrib.com/sltrib/outdoors/50260217-117/river-green-gorge-pipeline.html.csp [January 24, 2011]). The controversy in the title of the article refers to a plan by a Colorado developer to siphon off huge amounts of Green River water from Flaming Gorge and pump it to the Front Range of Colorado.

46. Russ Perry, telephone conversation, January 20, 2011.

47. "Penstock Modification Structures Tested at Flaming Gorge Dam," *Vernal Express*, June 29, 1978.

48. Many different hybrids have developed now in the Green River.

49. Russ Perry is one of those. A lifelong resident of Vernal, Utah, and avid river runner and fisherman, Perry wrote the original petition that helped to create the modern day blue-ribbon fishery but now no longer fishes there because of the competition. Russ Perry, telephone conversation, January 20, 2011.

50. Buzz Belknap and Loie Belknap Evans, *Belknap's Waterproof Dinosaur River Guide* (Evergreen, Colo.: Westwater Books, 2008), 14–17.

51. The information about fly fishing and its economic impact was derived from a telephone conversation with Steve Schmidt of Western Fly Fishers, May 19, 2011; and a telephone conversation with Nanette Gale, Ashley National Forest, May 23, 2011.

52. Johnson, *A History of Daggett County*, 219.

53. John Wesley Powell, *Exploration of the Colorado River and Its Canyons*, 247.

54. Cal Giddings, oral interview, July 3, 1984.

BIBLIOGRAPHY

Books

Baker, Pearl. *Trail on the Water*. Boulder, Colo.: Pruett Publishing Co., n.d.

Beckwourth, James P. *The Life and Adventures of James P. Beckwourth*. New York: A. A. Knopf, 1931.

Burton, Doris Karren. *Behind Swinging Doors: Colorful History of Uinta Basin*. Vernal, Utah: Uinta County Library, 2001.

———. *A History of Uintah County: Scratching the Surface*. Salt Lake City: Utah State Historical Society/Uintah County Commission, 1996.

———. *Settlements of Uintah County: Digging Deeper*. Vernal, Utah: Uintah County Library, 1998.

Chittenden, Hiram. *The American Fur Trade of the Far West: A History of the Pioneer Trading Posts and Early Fur Companies of the Missouri Valley and the Rocky Mountains and of the Overland Commerce with Santa Fe*. New York: F. P. Harper, 1902.

Clyman, James. *Journal of a Mountain Man*. Missoula, Mont.: Mountain Press Publishing Co., 1984.

Cosco, Jon M. *Echo Park: Struggle for Preservation*. Boulder, Colo.: Johnson Books, 1995.

Dale, Harrison Clifford, editor. *The Ashley-Smith Explorations and the Discovery of a Central Route to the Pacific, 1822–1829*. Glendale, Calif.: Arthur H. Clarke Co., 1941.

Day, Kent C., and David S. Dibble. *Archaeological Survey of the Flaming Gorge Reservoir Area, Wyoming–Utah*. University of Utah Anthropological Papers 65. Salt Lake City: University of Utah Press, 1963.

D'Azevedo, Warren L., and William C. Sturtevant, editors. *Handbook of North American Indians*, vol. 11, *Great Basin*. Washington, D.C.: Smithsonian Institution, 1986.

DeJournette, Dick, and Daun DeJournette. *One Hundred Years of Browns Park and Diamond Mountain*. Vernal, Utah: DeJournette Enterprises, 1996.

Dellenbaugh, Frederick S. *A Canyon Voyage: The Narrative of the Second Powell Expedition Down the Green & Colorado Rivers*. New Haven, Conn.: Yale University Press, 1962.

———. *The Romance of the Colorado River*. New York: G. P. Putnam's Sons, 1902.

Dimock, Brad, editor. *Every Rapid Speaks Plainly: The Salmon, Green, and Colorado River Journals of Buzz Holmstrom*. Flagstaff, Ariz.: Fretwater Press, 2003.

———. *The Very Hard Way: Bert Loper and the Colorado River*. Flagstaff, Ariz.: Fretwater Press, 2007.

Dimock, Brad, Vince Welch, and Cort Conley. *The Doing of the Thing: The Brief, Brilliant Whitewater Career of Buzz Holmstrom*. Flagstaff, Ariz.: Fretwater Press, 1998.

Dunham, Dick, and Vivian Dunham. *Flaming Gorge Country*. Denver, Colo.: Eastwood Printing and Publishing Co., 1977.

Farnham, Thomas Jefferson. *Travels in the Great Western Prairies*. Monroe, Ore.: Pacific Northwest National Parks and Forests Association, 1983.

Ferris, Warren Angus. *Life in the Rocky Mountains*. Denver: Old West Publishing Co., 1983.

Flavell, George F. *The Log of the Panthon*. Edited by Neil B. Carmony and David E. Brown. Boulder, Colo.: Pruett Publishing, 1987.

Flowers, Seville. *Ecological Studies of the Flora and Fauna of Flaming Gorge Reservoir Basin, Utah and Wyoming*. University of Utah Anthropological Papers 48. Salt Lake City: University of Utah Press, 1960.

———. *Vegetation of Flaming Gorge Reservoir Basin*. University of Utah Anthropological Papers 43. Salt Lake City: University of Utah Press, 1960.

Frémont, John Charles. *Report of the Exploring Expedition to the Rocky Mountains in the Year 1842 and to Oregon and North California in the Years 1843–44*. Washington, D.C.: Gales and Seaton, 1845.

Harvey, Mark. *A Symbol of Wilderness: Echo Park and the American Conservation Movement*. Albuquerque: University of New Mexico Press, 1994.

Hillers, Jack. *"Photographed All the Best Scenery": Jack Hiller's Diary of the Powell Expeditions, 1871–1875*. Salt Lake City: University of Utah Press, 1972.

James, George Wharton. *Utah, Land of Blossoming Valleys*. Boston: Page Co., 1922.

Johnson, Michael W. *A History of Daggett County: A Modern Frontier*. Salt Lake City: Utah State Historical Society, 1998.

Kolb, Ellsworth. *Through the Grand Canyon from Wyoming to Mexico*. New York: Macmillan Co., 1914.

LaRue, E. C. *The Colorado River and Its Utilization*. Water Supply Paper 395. Washington, D.C.: Government Printing Office, 1916.

Manly, William Lewis. *Death Valley in '49*. New York: Wallace Hebberd, 1929.

McDowell, Carma Potter. *Linwood Resurrected: A Town Buried under the Flaming Gorge Lake*. Privately published, 2008.

Morgan, Dale, editor. *The West of William Ashley: The International Struggle for the Fur Trade of the Missouri, the Rocky Mountains, and the Columbia, with Explorations beyond the Continental Divide, Recorded in the Diaries and Letters of William H. Ashley and His Contemporaries, 1822–1838*. Denver: Old West Publishing Co., 1964.

Murdock, J. Neil. *Early History of the Colorado River Storage Project*. Washington, D.C.: U.S. Department of the Interior, Bureau of Reclamation, 1971.

Nunis, Doyce B., Jr., editor. *The Bidwell–Bartleson Party: 1841 California Emigrant Adventure*. Santa Cruz, Calif.: Western Tanager Press, 1991.

Powell, John Wesley. *Exploration of the Colorado River and Its Canyons*. New York: Dover Publications, 1961.

Purdy, William. *An Outline of the History of the Flaming Gorge Area*. University of Utah Anthropological Papers 37. Salt Lake City: University of Utah Press, 1962.

Quartarone, Fred. *Historical Accounts of Upper Colorado River Basin Endangered Fish*. N.p.: U.S. Fish and Wildlife Service, 1995.

Reisner. Marc. *Cadillac Desert: The American West and Its Disappearing Water*. New York: Viking, 1986.

Sharrock, Floyd. *Prehistoric Occupation Patterns in Southwest Wyoming and Cultural Relationships with the Great Basin and Plains Culture Areas*. University of Utah Anthropological Papers 77. Salt Lake City: University of Utah Press, 1966.

Shearer, F. E., editor. *The Pacific Tourist: Adams & Bishop's Illustrated Trans–continental Guide of Travel, from the Atlantic to the Pacific Ocean*. New York: Adams and Bishop, 1886.

Simms, Steven R. *Ancient Peoples of the Great Basin and Colorado Plateau*. Walnut Creek, Calif.: Left Coast Press, 2008.

Sprinkel, Douglas A. *Geologic Guide along Flaming Gorge Reservoir, Flaming Gorge National Recreation Area, Utah-Wyoming*. Salt Lake City: Utah Geological Survey, 2000.

Stansbury, Howard. *Exploration and Survey of the Valley of the Great Salt Lake of Utah, Including a Reconnaissance of a New Route through the Rocky Mountains*. Washington, D.C.: R. Armstrong, Public Printer, 1853.

Stanton, Robert Brewster. *Colorado River Controversies*. New York: Dodd, Mead, and Co., 1932.

Stegner, Wallace Earle, editor. *This Is Dinosaur: Echo Park Country and Its Magic Rivers*. Boulder, Colo.: Roberts Rinehart, 1955.

Stone, Julius F. *Canyon Country: The Romance of a Drop of Water and a Grain of Sand*. New York/London: G. P. Putnam's Sons, 1932.

Sumner, Cid Ricketts. *Traveler in the Wilderness*. New York: Harper, 1957.

Talbot, Richard K., and Lane D. Richens. *Fremont Farming and Mobility on the Far Northern Colorado Plateau*. Museum of Peoples and Cultures Occasional Paper 10. Provo, Utah: Brigham Young University, 2004.

———. *Steinaker Gap: An Early Fremont Farmstead*. Museum of Peoples and Cultures Occasional Paper 2. Provo, Utah: Brigham Young University, 1996.

Tennent, William L. *John Jarvie of Browns Park*. Cultural Resources Series 7. N.p.: Bureau of Land Management–Utah, 1981.

Terrell, John Upton. *War for the Colorado River*. Glendale, Calif.: A. H. Clark, 1965.

Urbanek, Mae. *Chief Washakie of the Shoshone*. Boulder, Colo.: Johnson Publishing Co., 1971.

Van Cott, John W. *Utah Place Names: A Comprehensive Guide to the Origins of Geographic Names—A Compilation*. Salt Lake City: University of Utah Press, 1990.

Water Resources Bulletin (Feb. 1947). Washington, D.C.: U.S. Superintendent of Documents, 1947.

Webb, Bob, and Diane Boyer, *Damming Grand Canyon: The 1923 USGS Colorado River Expedition*. Logan: Utah State University Press, 2007.

Webb, Roy. *Call of the Colorado.* Moscow: University of Idaho Press, 1994.

——, editor. *High, Wide, and Handsome: The River Journals of Norman D. Nevills.* Logan: Utah State University Press, 2005.

——. *If We Had A Boat: Green River Explorers, Adventurers, and Runners.* Salt Lake City: University of Utah Press, 1986.

——. *Riverman: The Story of Bus Hatch.* Flagstaff, Ariz.: Fretwater Press, 2008.

Westwood, Dick. *Rough-Water Man: Elwyn Blake's Colorado River Expeditions.* Reno: University of Nevada Press, 1992.

Woolley, Ralf. *The Green River and Its Utilization.* Water Supply Paper 618. Washington, D.C.: Government Printing Office, 1930.

Zwinger, Ann. *Run, River, Run: A Naturalist's Journey Down One of the Great Rivers of the American West.* Tucson: University of Arizona Press, 1975.

Newspapers
Deseret News
Grand Valley Times
Green River Star
Salt Lake Tribune
Vernal Express

Articles
Bradley, George Y. "George Y. Bradley's Journal." *Utah Historical Quarterly* 15 (1947): 31–72.

"Folbots through Dinosaur." *Sierra Club Bulletin* 37, no. 10 (December 1952): 1–8.

Jones, Stephen Vandiver. "Journal of Stephen Vandiver Jones." *Utah Historical Quarterly* 16–17 (1948–49): 19–174.

Kelly, Charles, editor. "Capt. Francis Marion Bishop's Journal: August 15, 1870–June 3, 1872." *Utah Historical Quarterly* 15 (1947): 159–238.

Leigh, Rufus Wood. "Naming of the Green, Sevier, and Virgin Rivers." *Utah Historical Quarterly* 29, no. 2 (April 1961): 137–47.

Steward, John F. "Journal of John F. Steward." *Utah Historical Quarterly* 16–17 (1948–49): 181–251.

Sumner, John Colton. "The Lost Journal of John Colton Sumner." *Utah Historical Quarterly* 37 (Spring 1969): 173–89.

Thompson, Almon Harris. "Diary of Almon Harris Thompson." *Utah Historical Quarterly* 7 (1939): 2–138.

Webb, Roy. "Les Voyageurs Sans Trace: The DeColmont-DeSeyne Kayak Party of 1938." *Utah Historical Quarterly* (Summer 1987): 167–80.

Primary Sources
Aleson, Harry. "Notes on Green River Trip, 1951." Harry Aleson Papers (MSS B 187), Utah State Historical Society.

Beckwith, Mary. Journal (1956). Box 16, Folder 3, Otis Marston Papers, Huntington Library, San Marino, California.

Blake, H. Elwyn. "Boating the Wild Rivers." Copy in author's possession.

——. "Diary of H. Elwyn Blake Jr." ACCN 1407, Special Collections Department, J. Willard Marriott Library, University of Utah.

Burg, Amos. Postcards, September 6, 1938. Box 283, Folder 20, Otis Marston Papers, Huntington Library, San Marino, California.

de Seynes, Antoine. "A Journal of Antoine de Seynes." ACCN 1206, Special Collections, J. Willard Marriott Library, University of Utah.

Frazier, Russell. "Hurtling Hell's Half Mile." Box 68, Folder 1, Otis Marston Papers, Huntington Library, San Marino, California.

Galloway, Nathaniel. "Diary of the Galloway-Stone Expedition." ACCN 1936. Special Collections, J. Willard Marriott Library, University of Utah.

——. Papers, ACCN 1938. Special Collections, J. Willard Marriott Library, University of Utah.

Galloway-Stone Expedition. Collected Journals. Box 75, Folder 20, Otis Marston Papers, Huntington Library, San Marino, California.

Holmstrom, Haldane "Buzz." Diary. Copy in Box 283, Folder 12, Otis Marston Papers, Huntington Library, San Marino, California.

Kendall, Helen. Journal (1960). Box 358, Folder 29, Otis Marston Papers, Huntington Library, San Marino, California.

Loper, Albert "Bert." "Notes of Bert Loper for 1922." Box 280, Folder 24, Otis Marston Papers, Huntington Library, San Marino, California.

——. To H. E. Blake. July 7, 1940. Box 280, Folder 24, Otis Marston Papers, Huntington Library, San Marino, California.

Marston, Maradel. Journal. Box 126, Folder 6, Otis
    Marston Papers, Huntington Library, San Marino,
    California.
Marston, Otis R. "Dock." "Notes on Green River Trip,
    1947." Box 133, Folder 20, Otis Marston Papers,
    Huntington Library, San Marino, California.
McCullough, L. C. B. Journal. Georgie White Papers.
    MS270 S14 B7 F4, Cline Library Special Collections
    and Archives, Northern Arizona University.
Nevills, Doris. "Woman Conquerors of the Colorado."
    June 15, 1941. MS 552, Box 28, Folder 9. Special
    Collections, J. Willard Marriott Library, University
    of Utah.
Page, F. Lemoyne. "My Trip Down the Green River." 1926.
    ACCN 1407. Special Collections Department, J.
    Willard Marriott Library, University of Utah.
Reynolds, A. K. Notes. Box 288, Folder 1, Otis Marston
    Papers, Huntington Library, San Marino, California.
Sharp, C. C. "Notes on Colorado River Trip." Box 278,
    Folder 42, Otis Marston Papers, Huntington Library,
    San Marino, California.
Smith, Keith. "Recollections of Keith Smith of Linwood,
    Utah, as Told to His Daughter Susan." Unpublished.
    Copy in Special Collections, J. Willard Marriott
    Library, University of Utah.
Steurt, Marjorie. "Diary of Green River Trip—1955
    September." Box 219, Folder 21, Otis Marston
    Papers, Huntington Library, San Marino, California.

Woodward, Julius M. Box 278, Folder 4, Otis Marston
    Papers, Huntington Library, San Marino, California.
Woolley, Ralf R. "A Boat Trip Down Green River from
    Green River, Wyo.–Green River, Ut., July 10–Sept
    14 1922." Copy in author's possession.

**Oral Histories (Special Collections, J. Willard
Marriott Library, University of Utah)/Interviews**
Amburn, Barbara Williams. March 16, 2011.
Brinegar, Lee Roy. December 3, 2010.
Frost, Kent. July 7, 2003.
Gale, Nanette. May 23, 2011.
Gardner, Carol Lynn. January 24, 2011.
Giddings, Cal. July 3, 1984.
Hallacy, Mike. October 28, 2003.
Harris, Laphene "Don." March 14, 1990.
Hatch, Don. March 10, 1984.
Hatch, Ted. August 7, 2003.
Nevills–Stavely, Joan. July 8, 2003.
Perry, Russ. January 20, 2011.
Purdy, William L. August 28, 1985.
Reynolds, A. K. October 12, 2004.
Schmidt, Steve. May 19, 2011.
Sleight, Ken. October 21, 2003.

INDEX

Numbers in *italics* refer to photographs. Numbers in **bold** refer to maps.

Aleson, Harry, 58, 80, 90

Amburn, Barbara Williams, 37, 40, 49, 132–37

antelope (pronghorn), 7, 11, 12

anthropomorphs, 11, 116

Arch Dam Constructors, 107, 110

Archaic culture, evidence of, 9–11

Ashley, William, 15, 21, 27, 39, 48–49, 69–72, 77, 80, 113, 117, 123, 140n24, 146n5; and inscription, *16*, 16, 71, 72, 80, 141n33

Ashley dam site, 106

Ashley Falls, xvii, 6, 7, 16, 20, 49, 63–65, **66**, *68*, 69–83, *73*, *74*, *77*, *78*, *79*, *81*, **84**, 87, 91, 95, 99, 106–8, *108*, 110–13, 117, 120, 126, 127, 146n2, 147n32

Ashley's Crossing, 43

Ashley's Flat, 43

Bartleson–Bidwell emigrant party, 7, 9, 18

bears, 7, 9, 65

Beckwith, Mary, 38, 52, 110

Beckwourth, James P., 48, 49, 70

Beehive Point, 6, 54, 55

bighorn sheep, 7, 9, 111, 116

Bishop, Francis Marion, 57, 58

Black's Fork, 17–19, 22, 29, 30–33, *30*, 114, 116

Blake, H. Elwyn, 75, 92, 93, 104, 146n20, 149n5

Bradley, George, 64, 71

Bridger, Jim, 14, 15, 17, 18

Brinegar Ranch, 37, **44**, 117, 118, 142n24

Browns Park, xv, xvi, xvii, 5, 6, 16, 17, 21, 29, 41, 43, 56, 63, 64, 83, 87, 88, 89, 91, 97, 99, 106, 117, 118, 119, 139n5, 148n21

Buckboard Hotel, **24**, 36, *37*, 117, 124

Bucket of Blood Saloon (Linwood, Utah), 42

buffalo (bison), 7, 8, 12, 13, 18, 23, 48

Bureau of Land Management (BLM), 98, 118

Bureau of Reclamation, 103, *105*, 106, 112, 114, 117, 118, 129, 139n5, 142n24, 149n10

Burg, Amos, 76, 80, 94

Burton, Orsen, 90, 115

Cart Creek, **66**, **84**, 87, 99, 105, 106, 109, 110

Carter Creek, 5, 58–60, *59*, **66**

Civilian Conservation Corps (CCC), 54, 56, 139n5

Clyman, James, 5

Colorado River Compact, 103, 148n4

Colorado River Storage Project, xviii, 103, 106, 149n7

Comet (steamboat), 43, *43*

Crampton, C. Gregory, xvi

Crows, 12, 48, 140

Day, Kent, 8, 115, 116,

de Colmont, Bernard, 28, 34, 76, 94–96, *95*

de Colmont, Genevieve, 34, 76, 77, 94–96

de Seynes, Antoine, 34, 76, 94, 95, 141n1

deer, xv, xviii, 7–9, 12, 45, 50, 59, 60, 85, 101, 120

Dellenbaugh, Frederick S., 16, 48, 56, 57, 63, 69, 72, 80, 144n13, 145n44, 146n4

Dinosaur National Monument, xiii, 53, 121, 149

Driscoll, Elijah "Lije," 39

Dunham, Dick, 8

"Dutch John." *See* Honselea, "Dutch John"

Dutch John, Utah, 107, *107*, 118

Dutch John Draw, 65, **84**, 87

Dutch John Flat, 87, 89, 90, 101, 107

Echo Park Dam, 104–6, 120, 121, 149n7

eagles, xv, 8

Eagle Creek, *60*

Eisenhower, Dwight D., 106

elk, 7, 11, 12, 21, 59

"Fall of Cottonwoods, The" (poem), 131

ferries (over Green River), 18, **24**, 33, 37, **44**, **66**, 89, 97, 118

Ferris, Warren Angus, 13, 38, 140

Finch Ranch, 39, 118

Firehole Basin, 31, 32

Firehole Canyon, **2**

Firehole Towers, xvii, *31*

fish, 8–9, 10, 12, *113*, 114, 124–26, 139n10, 151n42

Flaming Gorge, xvii, 5–8, 10, 18, 20, 43, *46*, 46–50, 56, 75, 85, 109, 121, 127, 151n45; archaeological survey, 113–17, 150

Flaming Gorge Dam, xiv, xvii, xviii, 6, 8, 40, 86, 87, 99, 101, *111*, *112*, *116*, 139n10, 143n31, 147n5, 151n45; construction of, 105–28; dedication, 121; enabling legislation, 107–8; opposition to, 120–21

Flaming Gorge National Recreation Area, 124

Flaming Gorge Reservoir, xvii, xviii, 10–12, 17, 19, 57, 123, 125, 129, 139, 140, 144n8; features flooded by (maps), **2**, **24**, **44**, **66**, **84**

Fort Bridger, 15, 17, 19, 39, 59

Fraeb, Henry, 17, 18

Fremont Indians, 10–12; petroglyph panel, *114*; sites, 116

Frémont, John Charles, 3

French kayakers (Bernard de Colmont, Genevieve de Colmont, Antoine de Seyne), 27, 28, 34, 76, 77, 80, 94–96, 141n1, 142n14

fur trade, 7, 13–18, 48, 117, 132, 139; and rendezvous, 14–16, 18, 39, 117, 129

Galloway, Nathaniel "Than," 56, 72, *73*, 88, 146n14, 148n15

Galloway-Stone Expedition, *26*, 27, 30, 56, 73, 76, 80, 92, 103, 113, 142n8, 147n4,

Gardner, Terry Lynn Jarvie, 131

Giddings, Cal, 83, 127

Glen Canyon, xviii, 104, 109, 113, 114, 115, 117, 121

Glen Canyon Dam, xviii, 113, 120, 150

Green River (city), Utah, 123–24

Green River (city), Wyoming, xvii, xviii, **2**, 5, 19, 22, *22*, 26, 27, 36, 41, 76, 104, 118, 122, 139n5, 141n2, 144n8

Green River Star, 28, 36

Green River Suck, 7, 48, 51, 69, 70, 144

Harris, Don, 80, 82, *82*, 96, 106, 149n9

Harsha Ranch, **2**, 29, 35

Hatch, Bus, 53, 56, 70, 75, 80, 81, 94, 96, 106, 109, 110, 120, 147n6, 148n15, 149n9

Hatch, Don, 56, 120

Hatch, Ted, 109, 113

Henry's Fork, 11, 16–20, 27, 37–41, 43, **44**, 47–49, **66**, 89, 104, 107, 115, 117, 118, 129, 131, 139n5, 143n36. *See also* Williams Ranch

Hideout Canyon, 106

Hideout Flat, 6, 27, 54–56, 75, 77, 78, 103, 110, 139n3, 139n5, 144n25

Hill, Amos ("Hermit of Red Canyon"), 64, *64*, 65, 75, 145n49

Hillers, Jack, 57, 87, 88, 126, 147n2

Holmes, Emma, xvii, 32–36, *35*, 118, 142n15

Holmes Ranch, xvii, **24**, 32, *33*, 33–35, *34*, 95, 117, 118, 124, 142n14

Holmstrom, Haldane "Buzz," 50, 75, 76, 81, 94, 144n9, 148n16; inscription, 80

Honselena, "Dutch John," 87, 147n2

Hook, H. M. "Theodore," 8, 22, 23, 98, 145n45; death of, 63, 64

Horseshoe Canyon, xvii, 5, 6, 47, 49–52, *50*, *51*, 56, 103, 121, 127, 144

Jarvie, Alonzo, 118–20

Jarvie, John, 89, 97, 98, 118, 148n21

Jarvie Ranch, xv, xvi, xvii, 64, 97, 98, **100**, 145n45

Jarvies Canyon, 11, 64

Jennings, Jesse D., 114–17

Johnson, Lyndon B., 121

Kendall, Helen, 63, 96, 99

Kennedy, John F., 121, *122*, 123

Kingfisher Canyon, xvii, 6, 8, 47, 50, 53, 54, 56, 57, **66**, 121, 127, 144n19

Kingfisher Creek, 53, 54, 144n19

Kingfisher Park, 53

Kolb brothers (Ellsworth and Emery), 8, 27, 29, 30, 33, 35, 49, 55, 61, 70, 73, 92, 139n7

Lake O'Mahoney, 123

Large, Shadrach "Shade," 39, 118

Linwood, Utah, 27, 36, 40–43, *42*, **44**, 47, 52, **66**, 116–20, *119*, 123, 124, 127, 129, *130*, 131, *132–37*, 140n26, 143n34, 143n38, 150n32–33

Little Hole, xiv, 7, 88–90, *89*, **100**, 112, 113, 126, 147n5, 148n8

Lodore, Canyon of, 8, 21, 49, 57, 69, 98, 103, 123, 141, 148

Logan Ranch, **2**, 29, 142n5

Loper, Albert "Bert," 56, 60, 64, *74*, 75, 92, 104, 148n13, 149n5

Manila, Utah, 36, 89, 118
Manly, William Lewis, 19–21, 27, 69, 80, 141n31, 141n36, 145n2
Marston, Garth, 80
Marston, Otis Reeder "Dock," 35, 36, 51, 123, 142n18
Martin and Woodward ("two young men from St. Louis"), 60–62
Mexican Hat Expeditions, 38, 52, 79, 80, 96, 110
Mormons, 12, 14, 19, 27, 141n31
Morton, Al, 81
mosquitoes, xvii, 8, 16, 27, 37, 38, 54
Murdock, J. Neil, 101, 106, 149n10

Navajos, xiii,13, 117
Neilson, Ole, 41, 52, 53; cabin of, *52*
Nevills, Doris, 30, 79
Nevills, Norman D., *27*, 27–30, 35, 51, 53, 56, 79–81, 90, 96, 106, 141n2, 141n4, 147n27, 148n17
Nielson's Flat, 6, 52, 139n3

outlaws, 42, 55, 72, 89, 91, 97

Paleoindians, 9, 129
Pattie, James Ohio, 13
petroglyphs, 11, *11*, 114, 116
Powell, John Wesley, 51–52, 54, 64, 68, 122, 127, 140n30
Powell, Walter Clement, 63, 71
Powell Expeditions, 18–19, 22, *23*, 27, 39, 48, 50, 53, 57–58, 63, 64, *68*, 70–72, 87–88, 139n3, 141n36, 144n13, 146n4
Purdy, William, 7, 36, 65, 81, 114, 115, 117, 141n3

railroad, 21–23, *22*, 27, 29, 39, 42
Rasmussen, Minnie, 119, *133*, 150n33
Rasmussen, George, 119, *133*
Red Canyon, xv, xvi, xvii, xviii, 6–8, 10, 11, 21, 56–65, **66**, 70, 72, 75, 80, 81, 83, 85, *86*, 87–89, *88*, *89*, 91, 94–95, 97, 98, 105, 113, *116*, 121, 126, 127, 144n6
Red Creek Rapid, xv, xvi, 6, 21, 83, 91–99, *92*, *93*, *95*, *98*, 126
Reynolds, A. K. , 36, 77, 78, 81, 96, 110, 147n32
Reynolds, Adrian, 28, 29
Reynolds, Ellen, 147

Richardson, Frank, 57, 58, 145
Richmond, William, 56, 88, 147
Robinson, "Uncle Jack," 15, 17, 39, 118, 132

salvage surveys (University of Utah), 10, 36, 113, 114, 117
San Juan River, xiii, xiv, xvi, 75, 104, 113, 117, 149
Seeds-kee-dee Agie, 12, 15, 140n22
Sheep Creek, 5, 52, 54, 115, 144n19, 144n22, 145n26
Sheep Creek Canyon, *54*
Shoshones, 12–15, 18, 23, 28, 39, 129, 140n16
Sierra Club, 59, 110, 120, 121
Skull Creek Rapid, 6, 7, *62*, 62–64
Sleight, Ken, 60, 110, 113, 120, 123, 150n17
Smith, Jedediah, 5
Smith, Keith, 27, *40*, 41, 52, 117, 118, 140n26, 143n34; home, *132*; and suspension bridge, *135*, 139n5
Smith and Larsen General Store, *133*
Split Mountain Canyon, xiv, 49, 110, 144, 145, 149
Stansbury, Captain Howard, 25
Steward, John F., 57, 71
Stone, Julius F., *26*, 27, 73, 76, 79, 80, 92, 103, 142n8
Sumner, Cid Ricketts, 31, 59, 142n10
Sumner, John Colton "Jack," 22, 67, 71

Thompson, Almon Harris, 57, 58, 63, 70
Todd-Page party, 27, 65, 75, 92, *93*
Trail Creek, 11, 64–65, **66**, 75
Treaty of Fort Bridger, 15, 17
Trimble, Kelly, 104, 106

Uinta Mountain Quartzite, 6, 105
Uinta Mountains, 5–6, 10, 12, *32*, 47–48, 50, 56, 72, 141n3
United States Reclamation Service, 103
United States Geological Survey (USGS), 27, 28, 30, 37, 38, 48, 75, 82, 92, 103, 104, 106, 142n14, 149n5
Utah Power and Light, 103, 104, 142n14, 149n6
Utes, 12, 13

Vernal, Utah, xiv, 41, 47, 72, 76, 90, 106, 120, 145, 145, 147, 151

Washakie, 13–15, *14*, 17, 18
waterfowl, 8, 10, 12
White, Georgie, 63, 96, 97, 110, 111
wildlife, 7–9, 11, 12, 59–60, 77, 94, 114, 120, 127

Williams Ranch, 39, *40*, **44**, **66**, 118, *135*, *136*
Williams, Albert "Speck," 89–91, *90*, 97
Wind River Mountains, 5, 12, 15, 34, 45, 49
Woolley, Ralf, 37, 38, 48, 53, 59, 62, 64, 65, 75, 104, 106, 142n14, 143n29

Zwinger, Ann, xiii